Peptic Ulcer Disease - What's New?

Edited by Jianyuan Chai

Published in London, United Kingdom

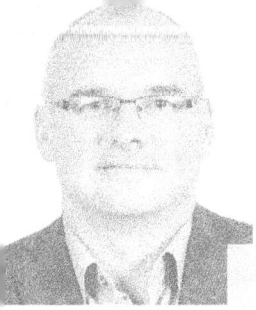

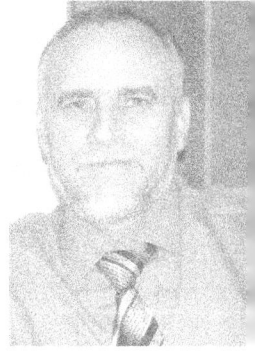
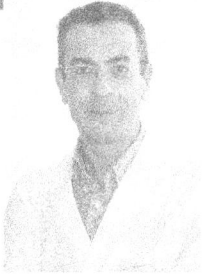
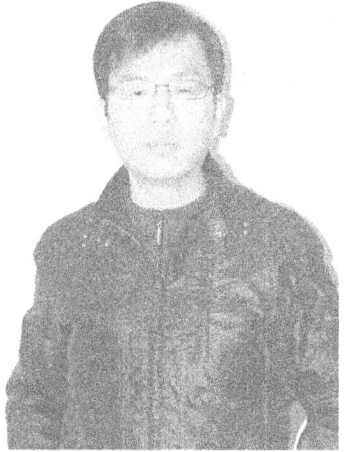
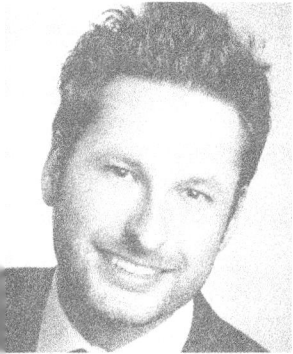
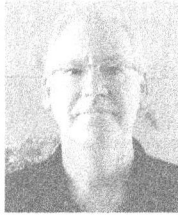

IntechOpen

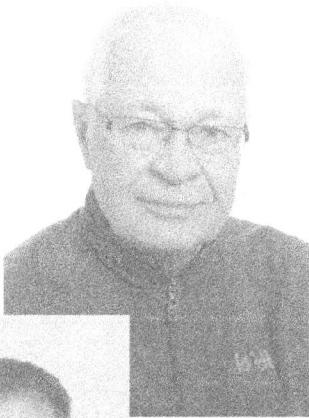
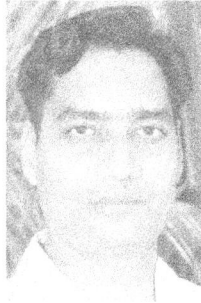
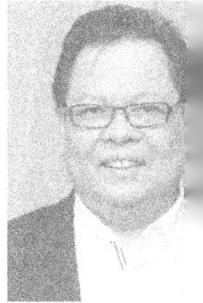
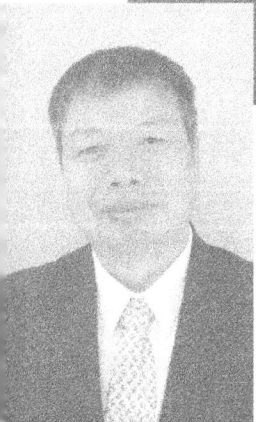
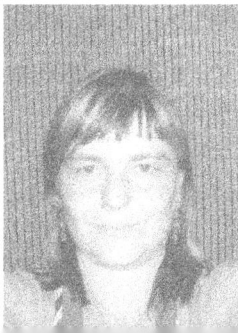
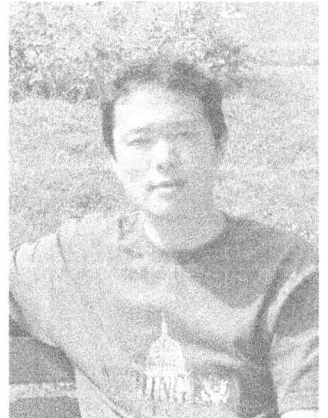

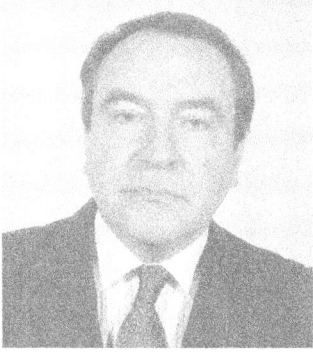

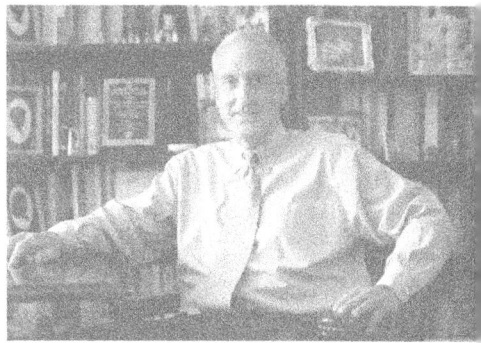

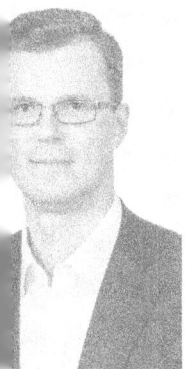

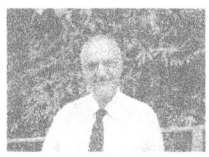

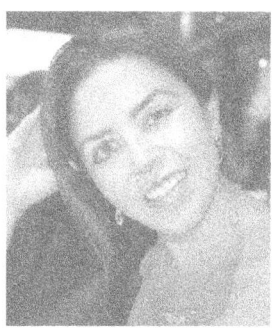

Supporting open minds since 2005

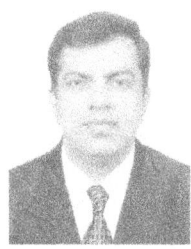

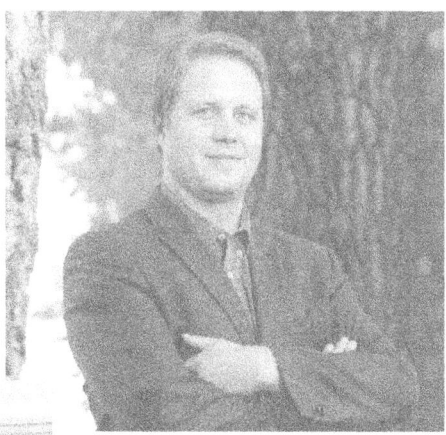

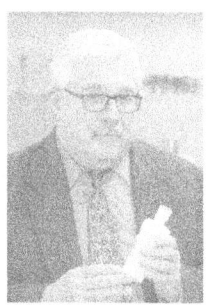

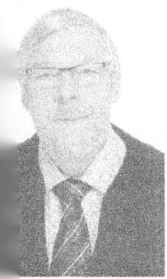

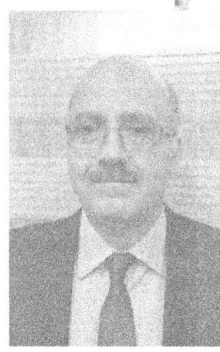

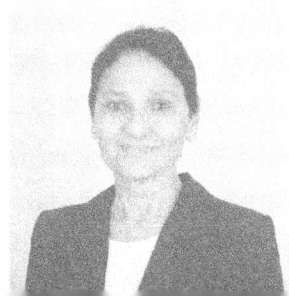

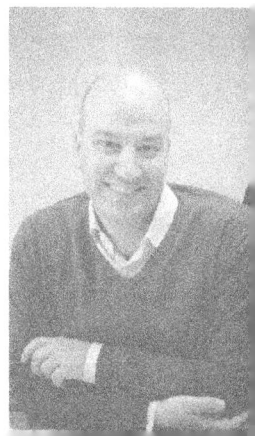

Peptic Ulcer Disease - What's New?
http://dx.doi.org/10.5772/intechopen.95182
Edited by Jianyuan Chai

Contributors
Carlos Casalnuovo, César J. Valdivieso Duarte, Pedro A. Bregoli, Carlos A. Vera Cedeño, Sampson Weytey, Annabel Barber, Gabriela Doyle, Cirlane Alves Araujo de Lima, Robson Silva de Lima, Jesica Batista de Souza, Ariel de Souza Graça, Sara Maria Thomazzi, Josemar Sena Batista, Charles dos Santos Estevam, Radu Seicean

Notice
Statements and opinions expressed in the chapters are these of the individual contributors and not necessarily those of the editors or publisher. No responsibility is accepted for the accuracy of information contained in the published chapters. The publisher assumes no responsibility for any damage or injury to persons or property arising out of the use of any materials, instructions, methods or ideas contained in the book.

First published in London, United Kingdom, 2022 by IntechOpen
IntechOpen is the global imprint of INTECHOPEN LIMITED, registered in England and Wales, registration number: 11086078, 5 Princes Gate Court, London, SW7 2QJ, United Kingdom
Printed in Croatia

British Library Cataloguing-in-Publication Data
A catalogue record for this book is available from the British Library

Additional hard and PDF copies can be obtained from orders@intechopen.com

Peptic Ulcer Disease - What's New?
Edited by Jianyuan Chai
p. cm.
Print ISBN 978-1-83968-419-7
Online ISBN 978-1-83968-420-3
eBook (PDF) ISBN 978-1-83968-421-0

We are IntechOpen,
the world's leading publisher of
Open Access books
Built by scientists, for scientists

5,900+
Open access books available

145,000+
International authors and editors

180M+
Downloads

156
Countries delivered to

Our authors are among the
Top 1%
most cited scientists

12.2%
Contributors from top 500 universities

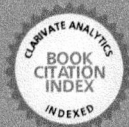

Interested in publishing with us?
Contact book.department@intechopen.com

Numbers displayed above are based on latest data collected.
For more information visit www.intechopen.com

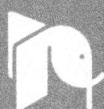

Meet the editor

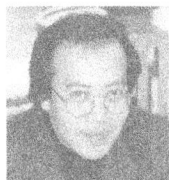

Dr. Chai received his Ph.D. in Biology from the City University of New York in 1998 and completed his postdoctoral training in molecular medicine at Harvard University in 2001. Then, he served the Department of Veterans Affairs of the United States as a Principal Investigator (2002–2016), in affiliation with the School of Medicine, University of California, Irvine. Currently, Dr. Chai is a professor at Baotou Medical College, China. He has published dozens of research articles on various subjects including zoology, cardio-vascular biology, gastroenterology, and cancer biology. He has been a member of the American Gastroenterological Association (AGA), American Heart Association (AHA), American Society for Biochemistry and Molecular Biology (ASBMB), and several other professional organizations and has served on the editorial board of multiple journals.

Contents

Preface

A peptic ulcer is a necrotic lesion penetrating through the entire mucosal thickness of the upper gastrointestinal tract. Although it mostly happens to the stomach, it can spread into the lower esophagus and the upper duodenum as well.

The cause of peptic ulcers is often blamed on either *Helicobacter pylori* infection or the use of non-steroid anti-inflammatory drugs (NSAIDs). However, although *H. pylori* infection is found in more than 50% of the world population, merely less than 10% of the population develops peptic ulcer disease. Furthermore, only 10% of peptic ulcer cases are found to have a connection with the use of NSAIDs. According to a 2013 estimate, at least one in five peptic ulcers have nothing to do with either *H. pylori* infection or NSAIDs use. So, what causes the rest of the peptic ulcers? Well, the reasons can be several. Topping the list is mental stress, which has been recognized as a contributing factor to peptic ulcers for many years. A typical example is a great earthquake that happened in Japan in 2011. The psychological trauma of this event led many refugees to develop peptic ulcers. Another factor is gastric bypass surgery, which is a common procedure to deal with the problem of obesity. About 5% of bariatric surgery patients develop marginal ulcers around the wound. Eating spiced food has also been connected to some cases of peptic ulcers. In addition, the concept of idiopathic peptic ulcer disease was introduced years ago. Zollinger-Ellison Syndrome can be such an example in which people are born with over secretion of gastric acid.

Nevertheless, all these factors have a common effect on the upper gastrointestinal tract, damaging the mucosal lining and exposing the epithelium directly to the highly acidic stomach fluid (~ pH 1–2). As early as the 1940s, scientists were learning through animal experiments that exposure of any living tissues to this fluid, including the stomach wall, is detrimental. The reason that our stomach or duodenum can normally tolerate such a hostile environment is the mucus overlaid on the surface of the epithelium, which shields the tissue from gastric acid. In addition, both the stomach and the duodenum contain cells that can produce bicarbonate to neutralize the acid intimate to the mucosal surface. When *H. pylori* dwells in the stomach or duodenum, it produces toxins that trigger the inflammatory response from the host, which can lead to mucosal atrophy, making the epithelial cells prone to acidic damage. Similarly, NSAIDs inhibit the production of mucus and bicarbonate, resulting in epithelial denudation. Therefore, the fundamental cause of peptic ulcers is stomach acid. As the German Protestant theologian Karl Schwarz said, "Ohne sauren Magensaft kein peptisches Geschwür," which means no acid, no ulcer. Anything that harms the mucus layer can potentially lead to peptic ulcer disease.

Peptic ulcer disease is probably the most common chronic infection in the human population. It had a tremendous impact on morbidity and mortality until a few decades ago when its connection to *H. pylori* was confirmed. Eradication of *H. pylori* infection has made a huge contribution to the decline of peptic ulcer disease. However, as mentioned, bacterial infection is only one factor. The final elimination of the problem requires more research on the mechanisms and a better understanding of the real cause. Despite many years of effort, peptic ulcer disease remains a major digestive disorder. According to the World Health Organization (WHO), each year more than 6 million people die of various digestive diseases; peptic ulcer disease is responsible for 4% of these deaths.

This book contains five chapters contributed by scholars from different parts of the world. Each chapter focuses on one aspect of the disease. Chapter 1 analyzes the causes of gastric ulcers and the auto-protection involved, including mucus secretion, epithelial construction, and the vascular, nervous, and immune systems built in the submucosa. It is a great inventory of what we are equipped with against stomach ulceration. Chapter 2 talks about *H. pylori* infection in young people. As we know, *H. pylori* infection is largely acquired at the early ages of life through various paths of transmission, such as contaminated food, groundwater, shared food utensils, shared personal items, and even kissing. This is true not only in developing countries but also in developed nations. It remains asymptomatic until later years in life. Despite the prevalence of peptic ulcer disease, it is rarely life-threatening unless complications develop, such as bleeding, perforation, or outlet destruction. In such cases, emergency care is needed. Chapter 3 gives detailed information on each of the complications, including how they are diagnosed and what are the right treatment options. It is a good reference for young clinicians. Chapter 4 elaborates on surgical treatment for peptic ulcers. Regardless of a bacterial infection or NSAIDs use or any other triggers, the fundamental cause of peptic ulceration is stomach acid. Therefore, acid-suppressive drugs are the first line of medication to treat peptic ulcer disease. Lastly, Chapter 5 compares vonoprazan, a novel potassium-competitive acid blocker, with commonly used proton pump inhibitors like lansoprazole and shows several advantages, including more effectiveness, fewer side effects, and more. However, it has not been approved for use in the United States or Europe. After this book is published, vonoprazan may be given a reconsideration.

Although we have been studying peptic ulcer disease since the medieval era (~ 11th century), today it remains a major digestive disease that troubles millions of people around the world. Needless to say, we have not done enough. We still lack adequate knowledge about this common disease. The aim of this book is to provide an update on the latest developments in peptic ulcer disease and inspire future research.

Jianyuan Chai
Baotou Medical College,
Baotou, China

Chapter 1

Gastroprotective Mechanisms

Cirlane Alves Araujo de Lima, Robson Silva de Lima,
Jesica Batista de Souza, Ariel de Souza Graça,
Sara Maria Thomazzi, Josemar Sena Batista
and Charles dos Santos Estevam

Abstract

Gastric ulcer (GU), a common type of peptic ulcer, results from an imbalance in the action of protective and aggressive agents. Gastroprotective mechanisms are mucus layer, gastric epithelium, gastric blood flow, gastric neurons, mucosal repair capacity, and immune system. Thus, the aim of this chapter was to provide an update on gastroprotective mechanisms. It was carried out through searches in PubMed covering the years 2016–2021 using several keywords. This survey resulted in 428 articles, of which 110 were cited in this chapter. It was reviewed the status of gastroprotective mechanisms and highlighted that mucins can act as a filter; gastric epithelial defenses are composed of the cell barrier, stem cells, and sensors on the mucosal surface; nitric oxide (NO) and hydrogen sulfide (H_2S) act for gastric blood flow homeostasis (GBF); the main effector neurons in the gastric mucosa are cholinergic, nitrergic and VIPergic, and oxytocin can activate neurons; repair of the gastric mucosa requires complex biological responses; the immune system regulates the entry of antigens and pathogens. The main knowledge about gastroprotective mechanisms remains unchanged. However, we conclude that there has been progressing in this area.

Keywords: hydrochloric acid, pepsin, mucus, gastric epithelium, gastric blood flow, gastric neurons, mucosal repair, immune system

1. Introduction

Gastric ulcer (GU) is a common type of peptic ulcer that stands out among different types of ulcers due to the frequency of occurrence in the digestive tract. In addition, it affects approximately 10% of the world's population [1, 2]. Although the number of deaths from GU complications has decreased in recent years, it still seriously affects the patient's quality of life and requires studies in this regard [3]. GU occurs as a gastric mucosal lesion that progresses to the lining of the stomach and becomes chronic and recurrent [4, 5]. In gastric ulcers, different stages of necrosis occur in the glands of the stomach tissue, participating in the formation process, neutrophil infiltration, reduced blood flow, increased oxidative stress and inflammation [6]. These changes are due to the imbalance between protective agents (e.g., production of mucus, bicarbonate, and prostaglandins) and aggressive agents (e.g., secretion of acid and pepsin) caused by different sources. People suffering from stomach ulcers report stomach pains feeling when eating, nausea, vomiting often accompanied by blood, high temperature feeling in the stomach, burning, and bloating.

The main causes of GU includes nonsteroidal anti-inflammatory drugs prolonged use, alcohol intake, smoking, ischemia, delayed gastric emptying [7], chronic inflammation due to exogenous factors, stress (trauma, shock, and burns), *Helicobacter pylori* infection [8, 9] and some dietary habits. When the stomach is exposed to adverse conditions, it tends to increase the production of acid and pepsin and to decrease the production of mucus and other factors that protect the gastric mucosa, which leads to epithelial damage.

The mucosal epithelial damage causes disorganization of the simple columnar epithelium, capillary blood congestion, edema, and necrosis of the gastric mucosa [10]. When the gastric mucosa is injured, there is a continuous secretion of reactive oxygen species (ROS) leading to lipid peroxidation and, consequently, to a decline in the antioxidant defense mechanism [8, 11]. Reactive nitrogen species (RNS) also participate in this process. Both ROS and RNS lead to ulcerative gastritis, stimulate macrophages, and increase the release of inflammatory cytokines [tumor necrosis factor (TNF)-α and interleukin (IL)-6] and nuclear factor kappa B (NF-kB) signaling [12].

The most used drugs for the treatment of gastric ulcers in the last 5 years are proton pump inhibitors (PPI), histamine H_2 receptor antagonists, and antibiotics eradication of *H. pylori* [13]. However, they cause several adverse effects. PPI can produce hypomagnesemia, cutaneous lupus erythematosus, osteoporosis-related fracture, acute kidney injury, and an increased risk of gastrointestinal infections [14]. Ranitidine can cause cancer in humans due to the presence of impurities containing N-nitrosodimethylamine [15]. Antibiotics, on the other hand, can develop bacterial resistance in users [16].

It is important to highlight that, although therapies with anti-H2 and PPI are already well established for the treatment of UG, they do not prevent its recurrence and may occur drug interactions in some patients [17, 18]. In view of these unfavorable properties, many researchers have searched for more effective and safer alternative anti-ulcer agents to treat GU that have less or no adverse effects [11, 17, 19].

Therefore, it is necessary to know the gastroprotective mechanisms which are essential to the development of new drugs for the prevention and treatment of GU. In general, gastroprotective mechanisms are mucus layer, gastric epithelium, gastric blood flow, mucosal repair capacity, gastric neurons, and immune system [20–25]. Therefore, the aim of this research was to discuss the gastroprotective mechanisms in the stomach and update the existing knowledge on the subject.

2. Method

This chapter presents an update on gastroprotective mechanisms based on research in PUBMED using the following words—gastroprotective action mechanisms (113 articles); gastric protection against hydrochloric acid and pepsin (4); function of hydrochloric acid and pepsin (31); types of pepsinogen in the stomach (16); function of gastric mucus and bicarbonate (7); gastric mucus and bicarbonate (9); gastric mucus formation (258); gastric sodium bicarbonate (91); defense of the gastric epithelium (43); blood flow gastric defense (15); vascular endothelial growth factor in gastric defense (4); gastric neurons mucosal defense (5); IL-1β gastric defense (16); stomach interneurons (9). A total of 428 articles were found on the topic researched between the years 2016 to 2021 and, of these, 110 were cited for containing relevant content within the scope of this chapter. The main approach of this update was on the gastroprotective mechanisms related to the prevention and treatment of gastric ulcers.

3. Gastroprotective mechanisms

3.1 Hydrochloric acid and pepsin

Increased production of HCL in the stomach leads to increased conversion of pepsinogen to pepsin. Together, these two substances can cause loss of gastric integrity and constitute harmful agents for the stomach.

The gastric juice is a liquid constituted mainly by HCl, lipase, and pepsin [26]. HCl acts actively in food digestion and is part of the protective barrier against pathogens ingested in food or water [27]. HCl is produced mainly by parietal cells and its secretion is stimulated by gastrin hormone in the gastric antrum G cells in response to food intake. Its secretion is mediated by vagal stimulation and gastrin-releasing peptides [23, 27]. In addition, other endogenous agents also participate in gastric acid secretion, such as histamine released from enterochromaffin cells (paracrine pathway) and acetylcholine from enteric neurons (neurocrine pathway).

Pepsin is the enzyme contained in gastric juice responsible for the digestion of proteins. It is produced by the main cells from the inactive form "pepsinogen" stored in zymogen granules. Under physiological or chemical signals, these granules secrete pepsinogen into the gastric cavity, where is activated into pepsin in the presence of HCl from the gastric juice [24, 28, 29]. The main cells secrete pepsin in its inactive form that prevents the self-digestion of protective proteins in the lining of the gastrointestinal tract. The pepsin activation only occurs in the presence of HCl [27].

There are two types of pepsinogens, type A (with three subtypes A3, A4, and A5) and type C [28, 29]. Other authors refer to pepsinogen as type I and type II. However, type A pepsinogen has characteristics common to type I and, type C to type II. Type I is formed by main gastric cells, whereas type II is formed in the fundic glands in the stomach, pyloric glands, and Brunner's glands in the duodenum [30]. Type I is reduced in cases of stomach mucosa atrophy below 30 µg/L, and type II can be secreted into the gastric lumen or the circulation, and its concentration in the blood increases in case of gastritis of different origins [31]. In another study, the authors found a relationship between gastric cancer risk and a low level of serum pepsinogen [32]. The diagnosis of atrophic gastritis of the body (AGB) is evaluated by the relationship between the pepsinogen I blood concentration and pepsinogen I versus II proportion (if < 3 means that the patient has AGB), whose values represent the mass of glandulocytes and the main glands in the body region of the stomach [31].

Pepsinogen type A can be used as a diagnostic biomarker for chronic atrophic gastritis and gastric neoplasms [33], and type C pepsinogen as a biomarker for prediction, diagnosis, and prognosis of different types of cancer because it has a broad-spectrum expression characteristic [28].

In a study to assess clinicopathological features of gastric adenocarcinoma of the fundic gland by endoscopy, 90–100% of clinical cases showed positive immunostaining for type I pepsinogen [34]. The honeycomb gastric cancer had negative immunostaining for pepsinogen type I/H+/K+-ATPase [35]. In another study, the authors reported that type I pepsinogen levels were found to be increased in individuals with gastric cancer and peptic ulcers affected by type I *H. pylori* (which expresses CagA and VacA type proteins) [30]. These authors argue that the different levels of pepsinogen found are probably due to the use of different methods of analysis or population of patients involved and, perhaps, it is uncertain to assess cancer risks and its progression by pepsinogen levels, which require other more accurate tests, such as endoscopy.

3.2 Mucus layer

The mucous epithelium promotes the internal protection of the organs in relation to the external environment (respiratory, digestive, urinary, and reproductive systems) [36]. In the stomach, the mucus-bicarbonate layer has a peculiar role, because it has gelling property and forms a physical barrier against the self-digestion of the epithelium by HCl and pepsin. It covers the mucosal surface and ensures acid neutralization, maintaining the basophilic pH [37–42]. Mucus is a viscoelastic hydrogel with a thickness of ≥ 1 mm formed mostly by mucin molecules produced by goblet cells [43]. It has an antioxidant and protective effect on epithelial surfaces against dehydration, shear stress, and infections [40, 44], and promotes the protection of the gastric mucosa in host defense against pathogens and gastric irritants [45].

The mucus barrier in the stomach is composed of two layers, a very adherent inner layer and a poorly adherent outer layer [46]. This barrier is formed by water ($\leq 90\%$), some salts, carbohydrates, lipids, mucins and lectins [46, 47]. The basic components of mucus are mucin glycoproteins (such as Muc5AC, Muc1, and MUC6) and lectins such as trefoil factor (TFF) 1 and 2 and *Griffonia simplicifolia* II (GSA-II), which bind to MUC6 and stabilize gastric mucus [38, 47–50]. It is noteworthy that mucins are mainly responsible for the viscous character of mucus and TFFs are typical constituents of mucus-secreting epithelia [28, 50, 51]. In gastric neoplasms with differentiation of the oxyntic glands, immature MUC6 is produced from the pyloric gland, with an absence of $\alpha 1,4$-linked N-acetylglucosamines glycosylation [52], MUC6 positive immunostaining occurs in gastric adenocarcinoma of the fundic gland [34] and MUC5AC/MUC6 positive immunostaining for honeycomb gastric cancer [35].

Mucus can be readily permeable to H^+ and HCO_3^- ions, preventing most HCO_3^- secreted by epithelial cells from mixing with acid, keeping the pH gradient almost neutral [38]. The hypothesis of hydrogen sequestration by mucus is as follows— hydrogen is bound to mucin polymers and the degradation of mucin polymers in the presence of activated pepsin would decrease the capacity of hydrogen sequestration [39], being released in the light of the stomach. On the mucosal surface, the pH gradient is almost neutral due to the retention of HCO_3^- [37, 47]. HCO_3^- is an inorganic alkaline salt that neutralizes excess gastric acidity. The conversion of CO_2 to HCO_3^- is catalyzed by carbonic anhydrase (metalloenzymes) at low pH and by hypoxia in the gastric mucosa [53].

To maintain a balanced pH gradient, HCO_3^- secretion must be in the same order of magnitude as hydrogen secretion according to a model based on the physics of ion transport within the mucosal layer according to the Nernst–Planck Equation [39]. In a neutral environment, mucus forms a tangle of polymers with adequate conformations for the passage of gases and nutrients and constitutes a lubricant against shear stress. Under acidic conditions, mucus constitutes a weak gel with adequate elasticity against gastric acids [41].

Mucins are high molecular weight glycoproteins that can act as a filter to prevent or delay the diffusion of harmful molecules and the entry of pathogens [44, 51]. If mucin production is altered and the mucus layer is damaged, infections such as *H. pylori* can occur [44, 45]. With a greater supply of water, there is a greater separation of mucin chains, as their density formed by interactions between mucins is reduced and may compromise their bactericidal function [41]. In this sense, adequate mucin production and balanced hydration promote the ideal structural condition against pathogen invasion.

Mucosal lining factors are directly involved in normalizing the gastric environment and GU healing [54, 55]. During the process of normalization of the gastric environment, the production of mucus can be stimulated by nitric oxide (NO) and hydrogen sulfide (H_2S) donors that interact with each other to produce mucus [56].

In ethanol-induced GU experiments, it is observed that in the negative control animals there is a reduction in mucus production, decrease in pH, and increase in gastric acidity [57]. After dissolving the mucus, ethanol inhibits the protective capacity of the mucosa, increases its permeability (allowing transport of large molecules) and leads to the dissolution of lipoproteins in the cell membrane [42, 57].

3.3 Gastric epithelium

The gastric epithelium is formed by a continuous layer of narrow junctions cells with secretory and digestive functions [57, 58]. The main cells that the infectious agent *H. pylori* tries to attach are the gastric epithelial cells [59].

Some of the protective mechanisms of the gastric epithelium include—cell barrier against the entry of toxic or pathogenic agents, stem cells that differentiate into gastric epithelial cells, and sensors located on the mucosal surface capable of detecting microbial antigens, leading to the induction of autonomic mechanisms that result in the effective killing of bacteria [60–62]. One of the proteins responsible for supporting the integrity of the protective barrier is β-catenin, acting as an adherent junction molecule together with E-cadherin [63].

This epithelial barrier is continually renewed by a small population of long-lived dividing stem cells; the renewal period is short, typically ranging from 3 to 10 days depending on your location [64, 65]. The generations of basal stem cells directly neutralize the colonization by pathogens by sensing their approach, promoting the regeneration of clean epithelial cells in the lumen [60].

In addition to the mucosa having cell renewal mechanisms for its own maintenance and secreting hydrochloric acid, pepsin and mucus under normal physiological conditions, it has sensors located on the cell surface that lead to the induction of the invader's death by autonomous effector mechanisms [60]. For example, when gastric epithelial cells become infected by pathogens, they produce factors that recruit immune cells, such as matrix metalloproteinases [66].

3.4 Gastric blood flow

Adequate gastric blood flow (GBF) is a protective factor for the gastric mucosa that has the primary role of maintaining its integrity [25, 56].

Gastric stress-related mucosal disease (SRMD) can lead to ulceration by compromised gastric defenses through gastrointestinal hypoperfusion and, subsequently, ischemia [37]. In order to repair the gastric injury caused by stress, angiotensin (1–7), a metabolite of the renin angiotensin system, NO, H_2S or carbon monoxide (CO) and ghrelin, nesfatin-1 and apelin peptides, participate; together, all these factors promote an increase in gastric microcirculation [67].

Among mediators that induce gastric damage are oxidative stress and inflammation [68]. Ethanol is the main cause of gastric damage in this regard, because it causes damage to vascular endothelial cells of the gastric mucosa, promotes hypoxia by increasing the production of ROS, induces the release of inflammatory mediators, and suppresses the activity of antioxidant enzymes [42, 69, 70], resulting in decreased microcirculation, submucosal edema, and development of hemorrhagic gastritis [45, 70]. Restoration of damaged blood flow in the gastric mucosa by ethanol requires removal of free radicals, pro-inflammatory cytokines, and inhibition of the transcription factor NF-kB-p65 [70–72].

Aspirin-treated rats have bleeding lesions in the gastric mucosa due to decreased mucus production due to cyclooxygenase blockade, inhibition of endogenous prostaglandin (PGs) synthesis, and decreased GBF [73–75]. The use of this drug also promotes an increase of almost 50% in the number of neurons that express the pituitary adenylate cyclase-activating polypeptide (PACAP), increasing gastric microcirculation [76]. In this sense, the resumption of the production of prostaglandins, as well as the increase in the endogenous production of CO and H_2S (produced by the enzymes cystathionine-γ-lyase/cystathionine-β-synthase/3-mercaptopyruvate sulfurtransferase or heme oxygenases) [75] and decreased number of PACAP-expressing neurons may contribute to the restoration of injured gastric mucosa and GBF. It is noteworthy that the interaction of NO and H_2S gaso-transmitters is very important for the maintenance of GBF and vascular homeostasis [77], as well as its restoration.

Other endogenous factors that contribute to mucosal recovery, as well as blood flow, will be discussed in the topic of mucosal repair capacity.

3.5 Gastric neurons

The main neurons present in the stomach are gastric interneurons and motor neurons [78].

The vagus nerve is responsible for stimulating the secretion of hydrochloric acid, and one of the first treatments for GU was based on severing this nerve in order to decrease acid production. Gastric neurons act on gastric motility, interact with hormones, regulate HCl and bicarbonate secretion, and induce immune responses [74, 76, 78, 79]. As an example of the interaction with hormones, oxytocin (OT) administered in the ventral tegmental area (VTA) can activate dopamine neurons in the dopamine pathway in the nucleus accumbens through OT receptors and improve the dysfunction caused by stress in the gastric mucosa, reducing the ulcer area, stimulating mucus production, and increasing gastric pH [80].

As part of the mechanism of gastric mucosal integrity, neuropeptides released by afferent C fibers sensitive to capsaicin participate [81].

Human gastric enteric neurons have been identified, mainly in the ganglionic plexus developed between the longitudinal and circular layers of the tunica muscularis called the myenteric plexus [82]. The main neurons identified were—with nonspecific dendritic architecture, cholinergic and nitrergic neurons; cholinergic type I uniaxonal spinous neurons are considered excitatory motor neurons or interneurons in the stomach; type I spinous neurons reactive to (NOS), and vasoactive intestinal peptide (VIP), considered inhibitory motor neurons and/or interneurons; and type II multiaxonal neurons (SOM), co-reactive for somatostatin. However studies are needed to assess the role of these neurons in gastric protection.

Among molecules that participate on the gastric ulcer defense mechanisms we can cite neuronal growth factor (NGF), PACAP, calcitonin gene-related peptide (CGRP) and NO. Reduction of NGF expression in gastric mucosa endothelial cells impairs endothelial cell viability, angiogenesis, and GU healing [74]. There is an increase in the number of PACAP-expressing neurons in the dorsal vagal nucleus in acetylsalicylic acid-induced gastritis, as described above [76], indicating that it is a factor in the neuronal response of inflammation in the stomach, acting to protect the gastric mucosa by reducing the secretion of gastric acid. CGRP and NO have a vasodilating action, probably participate in the mechanism of gastroprotection and increase in GBF in stress-induced damage to the gastric mucosa [81].

It is noteworthy that activation of the gamma-aminobutyric acid (GABA) A receptor of peripheral sensory afferent neurons in the stomach also appears to be involved in gastroprotection [83].

3.6 Ability to repair the mucosa

The integrity of the gastric epithelium depends on the maintenance of redox balance, antioxidant defense, and blood flow [65], as well as a constant renewal by stem cells. In this sense, the treatment of UG requires restoring the balance between cytoprotective agents and aggressive agents, either by reducing or neutralizing the production of gastric acid and/or stimulating gastric cytoprotection [84, 85].

During the healing process, there is a need for complex biological responses such as reduced inflammation, reduced oxidative effect, gastric cell regeneration, cell proliferation, migration, differentiation, gland reconstruction, granulation tissue formation, and neovascularization [3, 7, 86]. These responses are modulated by CO, glutathione peroxidase enzyme (GSH-Px), Cu/Zn superoxide dismutase (SOD), catalase (CAT), PGs, NO, sulfhydryl compounds, epidermal growth factor (EGF), vascular endothelial growth factor (VEGF) and the peroxisome proliferator-activator receptor gamma (PPAR-γ) [7, 10, 59, 75, 87–93].

CO is a gas molecule that helps to defend the gastric mucosa due to its vasodilating and antioxidant properties, improves hypoxia, and regulates Nrf-2 expression [75, 90].

The GSH enzyme is the main cellular antioxidant present mainly in the reduced form [67]. SOD and CAT enzymes are also important antioxidants [79]. These three enzymes constitute an important group of defenses against ROS that degrade gastric mucosa components and alter cell metabolism [45, 91]. Despite contributing to injury, ROS can reprogram differential cells together with antioxidant defenses (so that they are successful), as they can up-regulate molecules that stabilize and increase the activity of the cystine/glutamate antiporter, such as CD44v9 [92].

PGs are anti-ulcer agents that protect the barrier of damaged mucosa, increase blood circulation and bicarbonate secretion [67]. Increased production of endogenous PGs may result in increased gastric mucosal resistance against harmful agents, such as ethanol [51]. Particularly, PGs E_2 and I_2 amplify the secretion of bicarbonate and mucus contributing to the balance of gastric pH, maintain the blood flow of the gastric mucosa and coordinate the defense, renewal, and repair of the mucosal epithelial cells [45, 70, 93–95]. In addition, PGE_2 via the EP receptor can inhibit acid secretion and histamine release by parietal cells and enterochromaffin-like cells, respectively [95].

A study demonstrated that NO derived from inducible nitric oxide synthase (NOS) did not influence the healing process of gastric ulcers; on the other hand, the NO produced by the endothelial NOS isoform increased its healing [96]. NO acts as a gastric mucosal protector, activates K_{ATP} channels, modifies blood flow, neutrophil adhesion, and mucus secretion, and aids in wound repair [83, 89, 95]. NO and H_2S are small gaseous molecules that interact with each other, are freely permeable to the plasma membrane, and contribute to stomach homeostasis, integrating the control of mucus production, blood flow, mucosal defense, and gastric motility [77]. Endogenous sulfhydryls are also involved in the protective mechanism of the gastric mucosa [51].

Basic fibroblast growth factor (EGF) is responsible for the accelerated epithelial repair, increased mucus production improving the integrity of the gastric mucosa, and modulates the expression of cells called spasmolytic polypeptide expression metaplasia (SPEM) [2, 94, 97]. It is noteworthy that EGF and PGE participate as defense and repair factors of the gastric mucosa [96].

Vascular endothelial growth factor (VEGF) a functions to promote angiogenesis and protect gastric endothelial cells [74, 98]. Finally, activation of PPARγ protects against stress-induced gastric ulcer [86].

3.7 Immune system

The innate immune system can recognize molecular patterns associated with common pathogens in microbes and molecular patterns associated with damage through cell damage and the necrosis process through pattern recognition receptors [99].

Antimicrobial peptides form a chemical border between the epithelium and the mucus layer essential in the innate immune response to pathogen infection and are responsible for killing bacteria, fungi, protozoa, and viruses [61, 100]. However, if this chemical defense fails or the pathogen adapts and overcomes both physical and chemical barriers to reach the epithelium, the epithelial cells emit responses to the immune system and the immune system produces specialized defense cells. We can report some of these mechanisms described in the literature—macrophages form one of the first lines of gastric defense against *H. pylori* infection [101]; CD8+ T cells are present in the gastric mucosa and can act as a pro-inflammatory [66]; IL-17 and IL-22 are able to inhibit the growth of *H. pylori in vitro* [102]. The interferon 8 regulatory factor circuit (IRF)-8 and interferon γ (IFN)-γ forms an innate immune mechanism in the host's defense against *H. pylori*, which may promote Th1 differentiation, in addition to increasing the inflammatory responses of gastric epithelial cells to eliminate the bacteria [103].

CagA-dependent *H. pylori* infection contributes to activate the mechanistic target of rapamycin complex 1 in gastric epithelial cells; then, there is an increase in pro-inflammatory cytokines TNF-α, IL-1β and IL-6, CCL7, and CXCL16 chemokines, as well as an increase in the antimicrobial peptide LL37, exerting pro-inflammatory and probactericidal effects, inhibiting *H. pylori* colonization [59].

However, if *H. pylori* resists to these defenses and advances in its colonization, it can lead to ulcer and gastric cancer; which is quite common, since in most cases the infection can last for decades because the immune response has been unable to eliminate the bacteria, and long-term damage can lead to dysplastic changes and malignant transformations [32]. About 17.8% of the different types of cancers in the world are caused by infectious agents, including cancer by *H. pylori* that corresponds to about 5.5% of this total and over 60% of cases of gastric cancer [31]. *H. pylori* has a molecular mimicry between its lipopolysaccharide and the human Le group antigens, Le Type 1 (Lea and Leb) and Type 2 (Lex and Ley), allowing the bacterium to escape the host's immune system response [104]. Its attachment to mucus is mediated by the Lewis[b] antigen in MUC5AC and can also be attached to the mucosal epithelium; however, antigens can lead to alterations in the glycosylation sequence in mucins, forming epitopes on oligosaccharide side chains and contributing to aggressiveness and metastasis of gastric cancer [38].

After the gastric injury, there is an increase in the count of circulating neutrophils and a reduction in lymphocytes; the count of these cells or others that are part of the immune system are markers for GU [54, 71]. In a recent study for the development of vaccines against the pathogen Helicobacter felis, an infiltration of the antibody Gr-1 in the stomach induced an inflammatory response that led to the formation of CD4+ memory T cells (TRM) essential for protection [105].

In gastric injury, inflammatory cytokines IL-1β, IL-6, IL-8, IL-10, TNF-α, and the transcription factor NF-kB-p65 are present [70, 71, 94, 106, 107]. IL-1β and TNF-α are increased in ethanol-induced gastric ulcers [57]. IL-1β is considered a hereditary factor for gastric cancer; and, its reduction together with the reduction of TNF-α contributes to the restoration of the gastric mucosa [57, 99]. IL-6 activates neutrophils, macrophages, and lymphocytes at the site of injury, resulting in oxidative bursts and the formation of cytotoxic metabolites [89, 106].

Activation of the mitogen-activated protein kinase (MAPK) cascade and NF-κB transcription pathways is critical in several inflammatory and immunomodulatory diseases [108]. TNF-α induces neutrophil infiltration in the gastric epithelium and activation of NF-κB, increasing its own production, considered the main pro-inflammatory cytokine present during GU [103]. NF-kB regulates the transcription of IL-1 and IL-6 by activating neutrophils [45]. In addition to the transcription of TNF-α, IL-1, and IL-6, NF-kB can promote the transcription and expression of more than 100 target genes, which express cytokines and pro-inflammatory enzymes, contributing to tissue inflammation. In this sense, inhibition of NF-kB is considered the key to reducing gastric ulcer formation [42, 70].

Neutrophils can increase lipid peroxidation, releasing ROS as superoxide and hydrogen peroxide, delaying ulcer healing [91]. ROS secretions activate MAPK signaling in the gastric epithelium, which further activates NF-kB and Nrf-2, which can suppress the inflammatory response by increasing the antioxidant capacity in the gastric tissue [89]. Corroborating this information, the main antioxidants such as SOD, CAT, HO-1, gamma-glutamylcysteine synthetase, and GSH-Px are regulated by Nrf-2 [109]. Thus, it is noteworthy that Nrf-2 mediated HO-1 induction has cytoprotective, anti-inflammatory, antioxidant, and anti-apoptotic activities providing a therapeutic target against SRMD [107].

IL-10 acts as an anti-inflammatory cytokine, negatively regulating Th1 cell expression, class II MHC antigens, NF-kB transcription, and costimulatory molecules in macrophages [17]. Therefore, ROS inhibition and immune system improvement are related to the GU healing process [20], as well as the inhibition of the inflammatory cascade and down-regulation of the transcription factor NF-kB result in the decrease of neutrophils in the gastric tissue.

During wound healing, peptides from the TFF family coordinate the process of cell migration/invasion, angiogenesis, and immune responses [90]. Peptides TFF1, TFF2 and TFF3 are critical for gastric mucosa protection and damage correction [70, 110]. The TFF2 peptide is expressed in the mucus-secreting repair epithelial cell present at the edge of the SPEM ulcer, which coordinates immune cell traffic during repair [93].

Macrophages contribute to ulcer healing, secreting collagenases and elastases to break down damaged tissue and stimulating the release of cytokines, which stimulate chemotaxis, the proliferation of fibroblasts, and smooth muscle cells to build granulation tissue [91].

4. Conclusion

We present a brief summary of the main gastroprotective mechanisms of gastric ulcer. Analyzing such mechanisms is of great importance for advances in the studies of new drugs that aim to attenuate or prevent the actions of aggressive agents in the formation of gastric ulcers. We observed that there was a little scientific advance in relation to gastroprotective mechanisms, among which we can mention: HCO_3^- secretion occurs in the same order of magnitude as H^+ secretion for the maintenance of the gastric buffer system in the absence of food; oxytocin can activate dopaminergic neurons in the ventral tegmental area reducing stress-induced gastric ulcer; the main effector neurons in the gastric mucosa are cholinergic, nitrergic, and VIPergic; the cagA-dependent *H. pylori* infection that contributes to activating the mechanistic target of rapamycin complex 1 in gastric epithelial cells; infiltration of the Gr-1 antibody in the stomach induces the formation of CD4+ TRM cells essential for protection from *H. felis*; and that the main antioxidants SOD, CAT, HO-1, gamma-glutamylcysteine synthetase, and GSH-Px are regulated by Nrf-2.

Acknowledgements

The author wants to thank Coordenação de Aperfeiçoamento de Pessoal de Nível Superior (CAPES) for the finacial support to the research.

Conflict of interest

The authors declare no conflict of interest.

Notes/thanks/other declarations

The first author thanks her mother Genadir Alves Araujo for helping her with taking care of her 5-year-old son, Pietro Araujo de Lima Pedral, providing her the necessary time to dedicate herself to this research.

Author details

Cirlane Alves Araujo de Lima*, Robson Silva de Lima, Jesica Batista de Souza, Ariel de Souza Graça, Sara Maria Thomazzi, Josemar Sena Batista and Charles dos Santos Estevam
Departamento de Fisiologia, Universidade Federal de Sergipe, Cidade Universitária Professor José Aloísio de Campos, São Cristóvão, Brasil

*Address all correspondence to: cirlanepink@hotmail.com

IntechOpen

References

[1] Araruna ME, Silva P, Almeida M, Rêgo R, Dantas R, Albuquerque H, et al. Tablet of *Spondias mombin* L. developed from nebulized extract prevents gastric ulcers in mice via cytoprotective and antisecretory effects. Molecules. 2021;**26**(6):1-17. DOI: 10.3390/moléculas26061581

[2] Wang X-Y, Yin J-Y, Zhao M-M, Liu S-Y, Nie S-P, Xie M-Y. Gastroprotective activity of polysaccharide from *Hericium erinaceus* against ethanol-induced gastric mucosal lesion and pylorus ligation-induced gastric ulcer, and its antioxidant activities. Carbohydrate Polymers. 2018;**186**:100-109. DOI: 10.1016/j.carbpol.2018.01.004

[3] Wang S, Ni Y, Liu J, Yu H, Guo B, Liu E, et al. Protective effects of Weilikang decoction on gastric ulcers and possible mechanisms. Journal of Natural Medicines. 2016;**70**:391-403. DOI: 10.1007/s11418-016-0985-1

[4] Sudi IY, Ahmed MU, Adzu B. *Sphaeranthus senegalensis* DC: Evaluation of chemical constituents, oral safety, gastroprotective activity, and mechanism of action of its hydroethanolic extract. Journal of Ethnopharmacology. 2021;**265**:1-12. DOI: 10.1016/j.jep.2020.113597

[5] Barbosa JAP, Santana MAN, Leite TCC, Oliveira TB, Mota FVB, Bastos IVGA, et al. Gastroprotective effect of ethylacetate extract from *Avicennia schaueriana* Stapf & Leechman and underlying mechanisms. Biomedicine and Pharmacotherapy. 2019;**112**:1-10. DOI: 10.1016/j.biopha.2019.01.043

[6] Sánchez-Mendoza ME, López-Lorenzo Y, Cruz-Antonio L, Cruz-Oseguera A, García-Machorro J, Arrieta J. Gastroprotective effect of juanislamin on ethanol-induced gastric lesions in rats: Role of prostaglandins, nitric oxide and sulfhydryl groups in the mechanism of action. Molecules. 2020;**25**(9):1-8. DOI: 10.3390/molecules25092246

[7] Neto LJL, Ramos AGB, Sales VS, Souza SDG, Santos ATL, Oliveira LR, et al. Gastroprotective and ulcer healing effects of hydroethanolic extract of leaves of *Caryocar coriaceum*: Mechanisms involved in the gastroprotective activity. Chemico-Biological Interactions. 2017;**261**:56-62. DOI: DOI. 10.1016/j.cbi.2016.11.020

[8] Kwon SC, Kim JH. Gastroprotective effects of irsogladine maleate on ethanol/hydrochloric acid induced gastric ulcers in mice. Korean Journal of Internal Medicine. 2021;**36**(1):67-75. DOI: 10.3904/kjim.2018.290

[9] Lu S, Wu D, Sun G, Geng F, Shen Y, Tan J, et al. Gastroprotective effects of Kangfuxin against water-immersion and restraint stress-induced gastric ulcer in rats: Roles of antioxidation, anti-inflammation, and pro-survival. Pharmaceutical Biology. 2019;**57**(1):770-777. DOI: 10.1080/13880209.2019.168620

[10] Prazeres LDKT, Aragão TP, Brito AS, Almeida CLF, Silva AD, Paula MMF, et al. Antioxidant and antiulcerogenic activity of the dry extract of pods of *Libidibia férrea* Mart. ex Tul. (Fabaceae). Oxidative Medicine and Cellular Longevity. 2019;**2019**:1-23. DOI: 10.1155/2019/1983137

[11] Zakaria ZA, Balan T, Azemi AK, Omar MH, Mohtarrudin N, Ahmad Z, et al. Mechanism (s) of action underlying the gastroprotective effect of ethyl acetate fraction obtained from the crude methanolic leaves extract of *Muntingia calabura*. BMC Complementary and Alternative Medicine. 2016;**16**(78):1-17. DOI: 10.1186/s12906-016-1041-0

[12] Raish M, Shahid M, Jardan YAB, Ansari MA, Alkharfy KM, Ahad A, et al. Gastroprotective effect of sinapic acid on ethanol-induced gastric ulcers in rats: Involvement of Nrf-2/HO-1 and NF-κB signaling and antiapoptotic role. Frontiers in Pharmacology. 2021;**12**:1-15. DOI: 10.3389/fphar.2021.622815

[13] Li X-M, Miao Y, Su Q-Y, Yao J-C, Li H-H, Zhang G-M. Gastroprotective effects of arctigenin of *Arctium lappa* L. on a rat model of gastric ulcers. Biomedical Reports. 2016;**5**(5):589-594. DOI: 10.3892/br.2016.770

[14] Tonchaiyaphum P, Arpornchayanon W, Khonsung P, Chiranthanut N, Pitchakarn P, Kunanusorn P. Gastroprotective activities of ethanol extract of black rice bran (*Oryza sativa* L.) in rats. Molecules. 2021;**26**(13):1-13. DOI: 10.3390/molecules26133812

[15] European Medicines Agency (EMA). Suspension of Ranitidine Medicines in the EU [Internet]. 2020. Avaiable from: https://www.ema.europa.eu/en/news/suspension-ranitidine-medicines-eu [Accessed: August 11, 2021]

[16] Xie J, Lin Z, Xian Y, Kong S, Lai Z, Ip S, et al. (−) Patchouli alcohol protects against *Helicobacter pylori* urease-induced apoptosis, oxidative stress and inflammatory response in human gastric epithelial cells. International Immunopharmacology. 2016;**35**:43-52. DOI: 10.1016/j.intimp.2016.02.022

[17] Nascimento RF, Formiga RO, Machado FDF, Sales IRP, Lima GM, Júnior EBA, et al. Rosmarinic acid prevents gastric ulcers via sulfhydryl groups reinforcement, antioxidant and immunomodulatory effects. Naunyn-Schmiedeberg's Archives of Pharmacology. 2020;**393**(12):1-14. DOI: 10.1007/s00210-020-01894-2

[18] Baiubon P, Kunanusom P, Khonsung P, Chiranthanut N, Panthong A, Rujjanawate C. Gastroprotective activity of the rhizome ethanol extract of *Zingiber simaoense* Y. Y. Qian in rats. Journal of Ethnopharmacology. 2016;**194**:1-15. DOI: 10.1016/j.jep.2016.10.049

[19] Zakaria ZA, Zainol ASN, Sahmat A, Salleh NI, Hizami A, Mahmood ND, et al. Gastroprotective activity of chloroform extract of *Muntingia calabura* and *Melastoma malabathricum* leaves. Pharmaceutical Biology. 2016;**54**(5):1-15. DOI: 10.3109/13880209.2015.1085580

[20] Zhenga H, Chen Y, Zhang J, Wang L, Jin Z, Huanga H, et al. Evaluation of protective effects of costunolide and dehydrocostuslactone on 2 ethanol-induced gastric ulcer in mice based on multi-pathway regulation. Chemico-Biological Interactions. 2016;**250**:68-77. DOI: 10.1016/j.cbi.2016.03.003

[21] Karunakaran R, Thabrew MI, Thammitiyagodage GM, Arawwawala LDA. The gastroprotective effect of ethyl acetate fraction of hot water extract of *Trichosanthes cucumerina* Linn and its underlying mechanisms. BMC Complementary and Alternative Medicine. 2017;**17**(312):1-8. DOI: 10.1186/s12906-017-1796-y

[22] Boby N, Abbas MA, Lee E-B, Im Z-E, Hsu W, Park S-C. Protective effect of *Pyrus ussuriensis* maxim. Extract against ethanol-induced gastritis in rats. Antioxidants (Basel). 2021;**10**(3):1-17. DOI: 10.3390/antiox10030439

[23] Fatima R, Aziz M. Achlorhydria. [Internet]. 2021. Available from: https://pubmed.ncbi.nlm.nih.gov/29939570/ [Accessed: September 8, 2021]

[24] Heda R, Toro F, Tombazzi CR. Physiology, Pepsin. [Internet] 2021. Available from: https://pubmed.ncbi.nlm.nih.gov/30725690/ [Accessed: September 8, 2021]

[25] Salaga M, Zatorski H, Zieli'nska M, Mosinska P, Timmermans JP, Kordek R, Storr M, Fichna J. Highly selective CB2 receptor agonist A836339 has gastroprotective effect on experimentally induced gastric ulcers in mice. Naunyn-Schmiedeberg's Archives of Pharmacology. 2017;**390**(10):1015-1027. DOI: 10.1007/s00210-017-1402-3

[26] Martinsen TC, Fossmark R, Waldum HL. The phylogeny and biological function of gastric juice—Microbiological consequences of removing gastric acid. International Journal of Molecular Scienses. 2019;**20**(23):1-22. DOI: 10.3390/ijms20236031

[27] Prosapio JG, Sankar P, Jialal I. Physiology, Gastrin. [Internet]. 2021. Avaiable from: https://pubmed.ncbi.nlm.nih.gov/30521243/ [Accessed: October 26, 2021]

[28] Shen S, Li H, Liu J, Sun L, Yuan Y. The panoramic picture of pepsinogen gene family with pan-cancer. Cancer Medicine. 2020;**9**(23):9064-9080. DOI: 10.1002/cam4.3489

[29] Rao Y-F, Cheng D-N, Xu Y, Ren X, Yang W, Liu G, et al. The controversy of pepsinogen A/Pepsin A in detecting extra-gastroesophageal reflux. Journal of Voice. 2021;**21**:1-9. DOI: 10.1016/j.jvoice.2021.04.009

[30] Yuan L, Zhao J-B, Zhou Y-L, Qi Y-B, Guo Q-Y, Zhang H-H, et al. Type I and type II *Helicobacter pylori* infection status and their impact on gastrin and pepsinogen level in a gastric cancer prevalent área. World Journal of Gastroenterology. 2020;**26**(25):3673-3685. DOI: 10.3748/wjg.v26.i25.3673

[31] Loor A, Dumitraşcu DL. *Helicobacter pylori* infection, gastric cancer and gastropanel. Romanian Journal of Internal Medicine. 2016;**54**(3):151-156. DOI: 10.1515/rjim-2016-0025

[32] Song M, Camargo MC, Weinstein SJ, Best A, Männistö S, Albanes D, et al. Family history of cancer in first-degree relatives and risk of gastric cancer and its precursors in a western population. Gastric Cancer. 2018;**21**(5):729-737. DOI: 10.1007/s10120-018-0807-0

[33] Bang CS, Lee JJ, Baik GH. Diagnostic performance of serum pepsinogen assay for the prediction of atrophic gastritis and gastric neoplasms: Protocol for a systematic review and meta-analysis. Medicine (Baltimore). 2019;**98**(4):1-4. DOI: 10.1097/MD.0000000000014240

[34] Chiba T, Kato K, Masuda T, Ohara S, Iwama N, Shimada T, et al. Clinicopathological features of gastric adenocarcinoma of the fundic gland (chief cell predominant type) by retrospective and prospective analyses of endoscopic findings. Digestive Endoscopy. 2016;**28**(7):722-730. DOI: 10.1111/den.12676

[35] Yamada A, Kaise M, Inoshita N, Toba T, Nomura K, Kuribayashi Y, et al. Characterization of *Helicobacter pylori*-Naïve early gastric cancers. Digestion. 2018;**98**(2):127-134. DOI: 10.1159/000487795

[36] Khémiri I, Bitri L. Effectiveness of *Opuntia ficus indica* L.inermis seed oil in the protection and the healing of experimentally induced gastric mucosa ulcer. Oxiddative Medicine Cellular Longevity. 2019;**2019**:1-17. DOI: 10.1155/2019/1568720

[37] An JM, Kang EA, Han YM, Kim YS, Hon YG, Hah BS, et al. Dietary threonine prevented stress-related mucosal diseases in rats. Journal of Physiology and Pharmacology. 2019;**70**:3. DOI: 10.26402/jpp.2019.3.14

[38] Mall AS, Habte H, Mthembu Y, Peacocke J, Beer C. Mucus and mucins: Do they have a role in the inhibition of the human immunodeficiency virus? Virology Journal. 2017;**14**(192):1-14. DOI: 10.1186/s12985-017-0855-9

[39] Lewis OL, Keener JP, Fogelson A. A physics-based model for maintenance of the pH gradient in the gastric mucus layer. American Journal of Physiology Gastrointestinal and Liver Physiology. 2017;**313**(6):G599-G612. DOI: 10.1152/ajpgi.00221.2017

[40] Sidahmed HMA, Vadivelu J, Loke MF, Arbab IA, Abdul B, Sukari MA, et al. Anti-ulcerogenic activity of dentatin from *clausena excavata* Burm.f. against ethanol-induced gastric ulcer in rats: Possible role of mucus and anti-oxidant effect. Phytomedicine. 2019;**55**:31-39. DOI: 10.1016/j.phymed.2018.06.036

[41] Ruiz-Pulido G, Medina D. An overview of gastrointestinal mucus rheology under different pH conditions and introduction to pH-dependent rheological interactions with PLGA and chitosan nanoparticles. European Journal of Pharmaceutics and Biopharmaceutics. 2021;**159**:123-136. DOI: 10.1016/j.ejpb.2020.12.013

[42] Yoo J-H, Lee J-S, Lee Y-S, Ku S, Lee H-J. Protective effect of bovine milk against HCl and ethanol-induced gastric ulcer in mice. Journal of Dairy Science. 2018;**101**(5):3758-3770. DOI: 10.3168/jds.2017-13872

[43] Moura FCS, Perioli L, Pagano C, Vivani R, Ambrogi V, Bresolin TM, et al. Chitosan composite microparticles: A promising gastroadhesive system for taxifolin. Carbohydrate Polymers. 2021;**218**:343-354. DOI: 10.1016/j.carbpol.2019.04.075

[44] Kootala S, Filho L, Srivastava V, Linderberg V, Moussa L, David L, et al. Reinforcing mucus barrier properties with low molar mass chitosans. Biomacromolecules. 2018;**19**(3):872-882. DOI: 10.1021/acs.biomac.7b01670

[45] Bang BW, Dongsun P, Kwon KS, Lee DH, Jang M-J, Park SK, et al. BST-104, a water extract of lonicera japonica, has a gastroprotective effect via antioxidant and anti-inflammatory activities. Journal of Medicinal Food. 2019;**22**(2):140-151. DOI: 10.1089/jmf.2018.4231

[46] Lechanteur A, Neves J, Sarmento B. The role of mucus in cell-based models used to screen mucosal drug delivery. Advanced Drug Delivery Rewiews. 2018;**124**:50-63. DOI: 10.1016/j.addr.2017.07.019

[47] Heuer J, Heuer F, Stümer R, Harder S, Schlüter H, Emidio NB, et al. The tumor suppressor TFF1 occurs in different forms and interacts with multiple partners in the human gastric mucus barrier: Indications for diverse protective functions. Internationa Journal of Molecularr Sciences. 2020;**21**:7. DOI: 10.3390/ijms21072508

[48] Liu F, Fu J, Bergstrom K, Shan X, McDaniel JM, McGee S, et al. Core 1–derived mucin-type O-glycosylation protects against spontaneous gastritis and gastric câncer. The Journal of Experimental Medicine. 2020;**217**(1):1-17. DOI: 10.1084/jem.20182325

[49] Heuer F, Stümer R, Heuer J, Kalinski T, Lemke A, Meyer F, et al. Different forms of TFF2, a lectin of the human gastric mucus barrier: In vitro binding studies. International Journal of Molecular Sciences. 2019;**20**(23):1-13. DOI: 10.3390/ijms20235871

[50] Hoffmann W. Trefoil factor family (TFF) peptides and their diverse molecular functions in mucus barrier protection and more: Changing the paradigm. International Journal of Molecular Sciences. 2020;**21**(12):1-20. DOI: 10.3390/ijms21124535

[51] Carrillo W, Monteiro KM, Martínez-Maqueda D, Ramos M, Recio I, Carvalho JE. Antiulcerative activity of milk proteins hydrolysates. Journal of Medicinal Food. 2018;**21**(4):408-415. DOI: 10.1089/jmf.2017.0087

[52] Yamada S, Yamanoi K, Sato Y, Nakayama J. Diffuse MIST1 expression and decreased α1,4-linked N-acetylglucosamine (αGlcNAc) glycosylation on MUC6 are distinct hallmarks for gastric neoplasms showing oxyntic gland differentiation. Histopathology. 2020;**77**(3):413-422. DOI: 10.1111/his.14165

[53] Li T, Liu X, Riederer B, Nikolovska K, Singh A, Mäkelä K, et al. Genetic ablation of carbonic anhydrase IX disrupts gastric barrier function via claudin-18 downregulation and acid backflux. Acta Physiologica (Oxford, England). 2018;**222**(4):1-17. DOI: 10.1111/apha.12923

[54] Adenivi OS, Emikpe BO, Olaleve SB. Accelerated gastric ulcer healing in thyroxine-treated rats: Roles of gastric acid, mucus, and inflammatory response. Canadian Journal of Physiology and Pharmacology. 2018;**96**(6):597-602. DOI: 10.1139/cjpp-2017-0399

[55] Saremi K, Rad SK, Khalilzadeh M, Hussaini J, Majid NA. In vivo acute toxicity and anti-gastric evaluation of a novel dichloro Schiff base: Bax and HSP70 alteration. Acta Biochimica Biophysica Sinica (Shanghai). 2020;**52**(1):26-37. DOI: 10.1093/abbs/gmz140

[56] Lucetti LT, Silva RO, Santana APM, Tavares BM, Vale ML, Gomes PGS, Júnior FJBL, Magalhães PJC, Cunha FQ, Ribeiro RA, Medeiros J-VR, Souza HLP. Nitric Oxide and Hydrogen Sulfide Interact When Modulating Gastric Physiological Functions in Rodents. Digestive Diseases and Sciences. 2017;**62**(1)93-104. DOI: 10.1007/s10620-016-4377-x

[57] Monteiro CES, Sousa JAO, Lima LM, Barreiro E, Silva-Leite KES, Carvalho CMM, et al. LASSBio-596 protects gastric mucosa against the development of ethanol-induced gastric lesions in mice. European Journal of Pharmacology. 2019;**863**:172662. DOI: 10.1016/j.ejphar.2019.172662

[58] Qin J, Pei X. Isolation of human gastric epithelial cells from gastric surgical tissue and gastric biopsies for primary culture. Methods in Molecular Biology. 2018;**1817**:115-121. DOI: 10.1007/978-1-4939-8600-2_12

[59] Feng G-J, Chen Y, Li K. *Helicobacter pylori* promote inflammation and host defense through the cagA-dependent activation of mTORC1. Journal of Cellullar Physiology. 2020;**235**(12): 10094-10108. DOI: 10.1002/jcp.29826

[60] Sigal M, Meyer TF. Coevolution between the human microbiota and the epithelial immune system. Digestive Diseases. 2016;**34**(3):190-193. DOI: 10.1159/000443349

[61] Hartl K, Sigal M. Microbe-driven genotoxicity in gastrointestinal carcinogenesis. International Journal of Molecular Sciences. 2020;**21**(20):1-24. DOI: 10.3390/ijms21207439

[62] Ahluwalia A, Jones MK, Hoa N, Tarnawski AS. Mitochondria in gastric epithelial cells are the key targets for NSAIDs-induced injury and NGF cytoprotection. Journal of Cellular Biochemistry. 2019;**120**:1-9. DOI: 10.1002/jcb.28445

[63] Arita S, Kinoshita Y, Ushida K, Enomoto A, Inagaki-Ohara K. High-fat diet feeding promotes stemness and precancerous changes in murine gastric mucosa mediated by leptin receptor signaling pathway. Archives Biochemistry and Biophysical. 2016;**610**:16-24. DOI: 10.1016/j.abb.2016.09.015

[64] Wizenty J, Tacke F, Sigal M. Responses of gastric epithelial stem cells and their niche to *Helicobacter pylori* infection. Annals of Translational Medicine. 2020;**8**(8):568-578. DOI: 10.21037/atm.2020.02.178

[65] Cherkas A, Zarkovic N. 4-hydroxynonenal in redox homeostasis of gastrointestinal mucosa: Implications for the stomach in health and diseases. Antioxidants (Basel). 2018;7(9):1-14. DOI: 10.3390/antiox7090118

[66] Lv Y-P, Cheng P, Zhang J-Y, Mao F-Y, Teng Y-S, Liu Y-G, et al. *Helicobacter pylori*–induced matrix metallopeptidase-10 promotes gastric bacterial colonization and gastrites. Science Advances. 2019;5(4):1-14. DOI: 10.1126/sciadv.aau6547

[67] Brzozowski T, Magierowska K, Magierowski M, Ptak-Belwska A, Pajdo R, Kwiecien S, et al. Recent advances in the gastric mucosal protection against stress-induced gastric lesions. Importance of renin-angiotensin vasoactive metabolites, gaseous mediators and appetite peptides. Current Pharmaceutical Design. 2017;23(27):3910-3922. DOI: 10.2174/1381612823666170220160222

[68] Saadaoui N, Weslati A, Barkaoui T, Khemiri I, Gadacha W, Souli A, et al. Gastroprotective effect of leaf extract of two varieties grapevine (*Vitis vinífera* L.) native wild and cultivar grown in North of Tunisia against the oxidative stress induced by ethanol in rats. Biomarkers. 2020;25(1):48-61. DOI: 10.1080/1354750X.2019.1691266

[69] Chen H, Olatunji OJ, Zhou Y. Anti-oxidative, anti-secretory and anti-inflammatory activities of the extract from the root bark of *Lycium chinense* (Cortex Lycii) against gastric ulcer in mice. Journal of Natural Medicines. 2016;70(3):610-619. DOI: 10.1007/s11418-016-0984-2

[70] Yu L, Li R, Liu W, Zhou Y, Li Y, Qin Y, et al. Protective effects of wheat peptides against ethanol-induced gastric mucosal lesions in rats: Vasodilation and anti-inflammation. Nutrients. 2020;12(8):1-13. DOI: 10.3390/nu12082355

[71] Araújo ERD, Guerra GCB, Araújo DFS, Araújo AA, Fernandes JM, Júnior RFA, et al. Gastroprotective and antioxidant activity of *Kalanchoe brasiliensis* and *Kalanchoe pinnata* leaf juices against indomethacin and ethanol-induced gastric lesions in rats. International Journal of Molecular Science. 2018;19(5):1-25. DOI: 10.3390/ijms19051265

[72] Yang HJ, Kim MJ, Kwon DY, Kang ES, Kang S, Park S. Gastroprotective actions of *Taraxacum coreanum* Nakai water extracts in ethanol-induced rat models of acute and chronic gastrites. Journal of Ethnopharmacology. 2017;208:84-93. DOI: 10.1016/j.jep.2017.06.045

[73] Hernández C, Barrachina MD, Vallecillo-Hernández J, Álvarez Á, Ortiz-Masiá D, Cosín-Roger J, et al. Aspirin-induced gastrointestinal damage is associated with an inhibition of epithelial cell autophagy. Journal of Gastroenterology. 2016;51(7):691-701. DOI: 10.1007/s00535-015-1137-1

[74] Tarnawski AS, Ahluwalia A. Increased susceptibility of aging gastric mucosa to injury and delayed healing: Clinical implications. World Journal of Gastroenterology. 2018;24(42):4721-4727. DOI: 10.3748/wjg.v24.i42.4721

[75] Magierowski M, Magierowska K, Hubalewska M, Adamski J, Bakalarz D, Sliwowski Z, et al. Interaction between endogenous carbon monoxide and hydrogen sulfide in the mechanism of gastroprotection against acute aspirin-induced gastric damage. Pharmacological Research. 2016;114:235-250. DOI: 10.1016/j.phrs.2016.11.001

[76] Reglodi D, Llles A, Opper B, Schafer E, Tamas A, Horcath G. Presence and effects of pituitary adenylate cyclase activating polypeptide under physiological and pathological conditions in the stomach. Frontiers Endocrinology (Lausanne).

2018;**9**(90):1-12. DOI: 10.3389/fendo. 2018.00090

[77] Lucetti LT, Silva RO, Santana APM, Tavares BM, Vale ML, Gomes PGS, et al. Nitric oxide and hydrogen sulfide interact when modulating gastric physiological functions in rodents. Digestive Diseases and Sciences. 2017;**62**(1):93-104. DOI: 10.1007/s10620-016-4377-x

[78] Furness JB. Integrated neural and endocrine control of gastrointestinal function. Advances in Experimental Medicine and Biology. 2016;**891**:159-173. DOI: 10.1007/978-3-319-27592-5_16

[79] Gillis RA, Dezfuli G, Bellusci L, Vicini S, Sahibzada. Brainstem neuronal circuitries controlling gastric tonic and phasic contractions: A review. Cellulan and Molecular Neurobiology. DOI: 10.1007/s10571-021-01084-5

[80] Xiaogian HL, Zhang X, Wang Q, Luan X, Sun X, Guo F, et al. Regulation of stress-induced gastric ulcers via central oxytocin and a potential mechanism through the VTA-NAc dopamine pathway. Neurogastroenterology and Motily. 2019;**31**(9): 1-14. DOI: 10.1111/nmo.13655

[81] Czekaj R, Majka J, Ptak-Belowska A, Szlachcic A, Targosz A, Magierowska K, et al. Role of curcumin in protection of gastric mucosa against stress-induced gastric mucosal damage. Involvement of hypoacidity, vasoactive mediators and sensory neuropeptides. Journal of Physiology and Pharmacology. 2016;**67**(2):261-275

[82] Anetsberger D, Kürten S, Jabari S, Brehmer A. Morphological and immunohistochemical characterization of human intrinsic gastric neurons. Cells, Tissues, Organs. 2018;**206**(4-5):183-195. DOI: 10.1159/000500566

[83] Viana AFSC, Silva FV, Fernandes HB, Oliveira IS, Braga MA, Nunes PIG, et al. Gastroprotective effect of (−) myrtenol against ethanol-induced acute gastric lesions: Possible mechanisms. Journal of Pharmacy and Phamacology. 2016;**68**(8):1085-1092. DOI: 10.1111/jphp.12583

[84] Júnior EBA, Formiga RO, Serafim CAL, Araruna MEC, Pessoa MLS, Vasconcelos RC, et al. Estragole prevents gastric ulcers via cytoprotective, antioxidant and immunoregulatory mechanisms in animal models. Biomedicine and Pharmacotherapy. 2020;**130**:1-15. DOI: 10.1016/j.biopha.2020.110578

[85] Arunachalam K, Damazo AS, Pavan E, Oliveira DM, Figueiredo FF, Machado MT, et al. *Cochlospermum regium* (Mart. ex Schrank) Pilg.: Evaluation of chemical profile, gastroprotective activity and mechanism of action of hydroethanolic extract of its xylopodium in acute and chronic experimental models. Journal of Ethnopharmacology. 2019;**233**:101-114. DOI: 10.1016/j.jep.2019.01.002

[86] Elshazlya SM, Mottelebb DMAE, Ibrahim I, A.A.E-H. Hesperidin protects against stress induced gastric ulcer through regulation of peroxisome proliferator activator receptor gamma in diabetic rats. Chemico-Bioogical Interactions. 2018;**291**(153-161). DOI: 10.1016/j.cbi.2018.06.027

[87] Bueno G, Rico SLC, Périco LL, Ohara R, Rodrigues VP, Emílio-Silva MT, et al. The essential oil from *Baccharis trimera* (Less.) DC improves gastric ulcer healing in rats through modulation of VEGF and MMP-2 activity. Journal of Ethnopharmacology. 2021;**271**(1-9). DOI: 10.1016/j.jep.2021.113832

[88] Magierowski M, Hubalewska-Mazgaj M, Magierowska K, Wojcik D, Sliwowski Z, Kwiecien S, et al. Nitric oxide, afferent sensory nerves, and antioxidative enzymes in the

mechanism of protection mediated by tricarbonyldichlororuthenium (II) dimer and sodium hydrosulfide against aspirin-induced gastric damage. Journal of Gastroenterology. 2018;**53**(1):52-63. DOI: 10.1007/s00535-017-1323-4

[89] Liu J, Lin H, Yuan L, Wang D, Wang C, Sun J, et al. Protective effects of anwulignan against HCl/ethanol-induced acute gastric ulcer in mice. Evidence-Based Complementary and Alternative Medicine. 2021;**2021**(2021):1-14. DOI: 10.1155/2021/9998982. eCollection

[90] Kwiecien S, Magierowka K, Magierowski M, Surmiak M, Hubalewska M, Paido R, et al. Role of sensory afferent nerves, lipid peroxidation and antioxidative enzymes in the carbon monoxide-induced gastroprotection against stress ulcerogenesis. Journal of Physiology and Pharmacology. 2016;**67**(5):717-729

[91] Adeniyi OS, Makinde OV, Friday ET, Olaleve SB. Effects of quinine on gastric ulcer healing in Wistar rats. Journal of Complementary and Integrative Medicine. 2017;**14**(4):1-11. DOI: 10.1515/jcim-2016-0132

[92] Meyer AR, Engevik AC, Willet S, Williams JA, Zou Y, Massion PP, et al. Cystine/glutamate antiporter (xCT) is required for chief cell plasticity after gastric injury. Cellular and Molecular Gastroenterology and Hepatology. 2019;**8**(3):379-405. DOI: 10.1016/j.jcmgh.2019.04.015

[93] Balogun ME, Besong EE, Obimma N, Mbamalu OS, Diobissie FSA. Protective roles of *Vigna subterrânea* (Bambara nut) in rats with aspirin-induced gastric mucosal injury. Journal of Integrative Medicine. 2018;**16**:342-349. DOI: 10.1016/j.joim.2018.07.004

[94] Chen W, Wu D, Jin Y, Li Q, Liu Y, Qiao X, et al. Pre-protective effect of polysaccharides purified from *Hericium erinaceus* against ethanol-induced gastric mucosal injury in rats. International Journal of Biological Macromolecules. 2020;**159**:948-956. DOI: 10.1016/j.ijbiomac.2020.05.163

[95] Moawad H, Awdan SAE, Sallam NA, El-Eraky W, Alkhawlani MA. Gastroprotective effect of cilostazol against ethanol- and pylorus ligation-induced gastric lesions in rats. Naunyn-Schmiedeberg's Archives of Pharmacology. 2019;**392**(12):1605-1616. DOI: 10.1007/s00210-019-01699-y

[96] Lebda MA, El-Far AH, Noreldin AE, Elewa YHA, Jaouni SKA, Mousa AS. Protective effects of miswak (*Salvadora persica*) against experimentally induced gastric ulcers in rats. Oxidate Medicine and Cellular Longevity. 2018;**2018**:1-14. DOI: 10.1155/2018/6703296

[97] Teal E, Dua-Awereh M, Hirshorn ST, Zavros Y. Role of metaplasia during gastric regeneration. American Journal Physiology Cell Physiology. 2020;**319**(6):C947-C954. DOI: 10.1152/ajpcell.00415.2019

[98] Cuzziol CI, Castanhole-Nunes MMU, Pavarino EC, Goloni-Bertollo EM. MicroRNAs as regulators of VEGFA and NFE2L2 in câncer. Gene. 2020;**759**:1-19. DOI: 10.1016/j.gene.2020.144994

[99] Cao X, Xu J. Insights into inflammasome and its research advances in câncer. Tumori Journal. 2019;**105**(6):456-464. DOI: 10.1177/03008916198680007

[100] Padra M, Benktander J, Robinson K, Lindén SK. Carbohydrate-dependent and antimicrobial peptide defence mechanisms against *Helicobacter pylori* infections. Current Topics in Microbiology and Immunology. 2019;**421**:179-207. DOI: 10.1007/978-3-030-15138-6_8

[101] Latour YL, Gobert AP, Wilson KT. The role of polyamines in the regulation

of macrophage polarization and function. Amino Acids. 2020;**52**(2):151-160. DOI: 10.1007/s00726-019-02719-0

[102] Dixon BREA, Radin JN, Piazuelo MB, Contreras DC, Algood HMS. IL-17a and IL-22 induce expression of antimicrobials in gastrointestinal epithelial cells and may contribute to epithelial cell defense against *Helicobacter pylori*. PLoS One. 2016;**11**(2):1-19. DOI: 10.1371/journal.pone.0148514

[103] Yan M, Wang H, Sun J, Liao W, Li P, Zhu Y, et al. Cutting edge: Expression of IRF8 in gastric epithelial cells confers protective innate immunity against *Helicobacter pylori* infection. The Journal of Immunology. 2016;**196**(5):1999-2003. DOI: 10.4049/jimmunol.1500766

[104] Fagoonee S, Pellicano R. *Helicobacter pylori*: Molecular basis for colonization and survival in gastric environment and resistance to antibiotics. A short review. Infectious Disease (Londs). 2019;**51**(6):399-408. DOI: 10.1080/23744235.2019.1588472

[105] Hu C, Liu W, Xu N, Huang A, Zhang Z, Fan M, et al. Silk fibroin hydrogel as mucosal vaccine carrier: Induction of gastric CD4+TRM cells mediated by inflammatory response induces optimal immune protection against *Helicobacter felis*. Emerging and Infections. 2020;**9**(1):2289-2302. DOI: 10.1080/22221751.2020.1830719

[106] Souza MC, Vieira AJ, Beserra FP, Pellizzon CH, Nóbrega RH, Rozza AL. Gastroprotective effect of limonene in rats: Influence on oxidative stress, inflammation and gene expression. Phytomedicine. 2019;**53**:37-42. DOI: 10.1016/j.phymed.2018.09.027

[107] An JM, Kim E, Lee HJ, Park MH, Son DJ, Hahm KB. Dolichos lablab L. extracts as pharmanutrient for stress-related mucosal disease in rat stomach.

Journal of Clinical Biochemistry Nutrition. 2020;**67**(1):89-101. DOI: 10.3164/jcbn.20-11

[108] Zhang C, Gao F, Gan S, He Y, Chen Z, Liu X, et al. Chemical characterization and gastroprotective effect of an isolated polysaccharide fraction from *Bletilla striata* against ethanol-induced acute gastric ulcer. Food and Chemical Toxicology. 2019;**131**:1-37. DOI: 10.1016/j.fct.2019.05.047

[109] Wu Y, Chen H, Zou Y, Yi R, Um J, Zhao X. *Lactobacillus plantarum* HFY09 alleviates alcohol-induced gastric ulcers in mice via an anti-oxidative mechanism. Journal of Food Biochemistry. 2021;**45**(5):1-9. DOI: 10.1111/jfbc.13726

[110] He H, Feng M, Xu H, Li X, He Y, Qin H, et al. Total triterpenoids from the fruits of *Chaenomeles speciosa* exerted gastroprotective activities on indomethacin-induced gastric damage via modulating microRNA-423-5p-mediated TFF/NAG-1 and apoptotic pathways. Food and Function. 2020;**11**(1):662-679. DOI: 10.1039/c9fo02322d

Chapter 2

Helicobacter pylori Infection in Peptic Ulcer Disease among Young People

Sampson Weytey

Abstract

Peptic Ulcer Disease (PUD) is a common chronic disease of the Gastrointestinal Tract (GIT) worldwide, affecting 87.4 million people with 257,500 mortality turnouts in the year 2015. PUD is a painful open sore that develops in the wall lining of the lower part of the esophagus, the stomach, or the duodenum. PUD has both internal and external causative factors, of which *Helicobacter pylori* (*H. pylori*) is a major role player, accounting for 70–95% of its prevalence rate globally. *H. pylori* infection is acquired generally during the younger ages of life with its various mode of transmission, and with a prevalence rate of 90% in some developing countries, but remains asymptomatic till later years in life. This chapter attempts to provide the overview of *H. pylori* infection among young people, since they differ from the elderly, in terms of its prevalence rate, its risk factors, its complication rate, its diagnostic tests and managements, and its higher rate of antibiotic resistance.

Keywords: *Helicobacter pylori*, infection, peptic ulcer, young people, asymptomatic, antibiotic resistance

1. Introduction

1.1 Background

H. pylori (*H. pylori*) seems to play a significant role in the development of Peptic ulcer disease (PUD), a disease which is said to affect more that 10% of the world's population [1]. From the global perspective, *H. pylori* infection affects above 50% of the world's population, and is known to affect at least one-third of the young people especially children [2, 3]. Up to 90% of the children in the developing countries get infected by *H. pylori* where as in the developed countries it has 1.8–65% prevalence rate [4]. In some parts of Africa, *H. pylori* infection rate ranges from 40–90% [4]. Most of the individuals according to knowledge from literature shows that nearly 10% of the children in the developing nations remain asymptomatic after acquiring *H. pylori* infection [5].

H. pylori is a gram-negative microaerophilic bacterium that affect the mucous lining of the stomach, especially the antrum [6, 7]. *H. pylori* infection may result in either developing gastric ulcer (70–90%) or duodenal ulcer (90%) or both [1, 8]. *H. pylori* infection occurs in the early stages of life, but remains asymptomatic, and can live with the affected individual for a long period of time until it is treated [7]. Common signs and symptoms identified with the infection among the young people includes nausea, vomiting, gnawing or burning abdominal pain, intestinal bleeding, gastric reflex, occasional fever, poor appetite, bloating abdomen, frequent burping, tiredness and weakness, and weight loss [5]. The effects of this infection can progress to more complicated form, causing both gastric and extra-gastric conditions if not treated early or left untreated [9]. *H. pylori* infection causes gastric adenocarcinoma through a progressive sequence of gastritis to atrophy, then intestinal metaplasia, then to dysplasia, and finally to carcinoma [10]. Several gastro-duodenal complications may develop once *H. pylori* infection is well established [11].

Literature shows that there are both invasive and non-invasive diagnostic investigations that can be used to determine the presence of the infection [2, 12]. The recommended management approach is the screen-and-treat strategies [3]. Usually, the first line of treatment is the triple therapy, and according to researched work has proven to be the best in the management of *H. pylori* infection among the young people [13]. It has been observed that clarithromycin resistance is the main cause of treatment failure among the affected individuals [14]. Due to the increased rate of antibiotic resistance in the eradication of *H. pylori*, recommendations have been made for the development, and the use of new vaccines to prevent the infection among young people [13, 14]. Research seems to prove that the infection of *H. pylori* increases with age, and the rate of infection among the elderly is higher than the youngsters, therefore critical attention must be given to children since 80% of the infection usually occur in childhood which usually persist until adulthood [7].

2. Bacteriology

H. pylori bacterium was first discovered by Marshall and Warren in the year 1983 after they have cultured a gastric biopsy specimen of Peptic ulcer disease patients over a prolonged period of time [15]. This bacterium initially was called Campylobacter until the year 1989, when it was given its currently known name when a sequence of ribosomal features revealed its uniqueness [16]. This essential gastro-enterological transforming effort gained global recognition and so won a Noble prize in physiology and medicine in the year 2005 [17]. Literature currently reveals the identification of about 22 more species possessing similar cellular morphology, and test positive for oxidase, catalase and urease test, and in addition have the stomach, and the intestine as their colonizing site in their mammalian host [2].

H. pylori is a helical-shaped, unipolar, multiflagellate, slow growing, micro-aerophilic, Gram-negative motile bacterium [7]. This bacterium typically is 0.5 to 1.0 μm in width, and can be 2.5 to 5 μm long [17]. *H. pylori* possesses smooth and round end surface from which evolves one to six polar-sheath flagella [18]. Age, growth conditions, and specie type can cause the spiral wavelength of the organism to vary [17]. Chocolate agar or blood agar are none selective agar media, and selective agars like Skirrow's brooded in a humidifier, micro-aerobic of 5% oxygen at the degree centigrade of 35 to 37, are some media agars on which the bacterium *H. pylori* can be cultured for 3 to 7 days [2]. It has been found that old, stressed or mal-nutritious and prolong air exposure of cultured cells can become idle or inactive coccoid which enhances its survival in feces, and even in water outside of the human host [17].

Irrespective of the hostile condition of the human stomach, *H. pylori* has the ability to colonize a specific biological micro niche within the gastric lumen, survive, and persist for a long period of time, if not treated effectively as compared to other microorganisms that thrives well in very low pH environment [7, 12, 15]. Research has proofed that *H. pylori* is mostly observed to be attached to the superficial epithelial cells of the gastric mucous layer without serious invasion of the stomach tissues of its host [13]. There are various essential features possessed by *H. pylori* that efficiently enhance its survival in the acidic condition of the stomach, causing infection [13]. This disease-causing microorganism uses its unipolar flagella to establish colonization, penetrate, and make significant movements between two regions of the stomach avoiding its acidic pressure [7, 15]. Studies have shown that *H. pylori* can cause significant interference to the human host's antigen presenting process, and subvert the pattern recognition of the innate and adapted immunity [15]. *H. pylori* can also thrive undisturbed by the acidic content of the stomach by secreting urease, which is able to set a conducive pH environment of 4–8.5 for its survival [15].

3. Epidermiology

H. pylori infection is among the world's commonest health problem, having more than 50% victims of the global population [7]. Epidemiological studies have revealed the fact that *H. pylori* infection prevalence is directly associated with its high incidence rate and long-term existence [2]. *H. pylori* infection compared with other related infectious disease has a high prevalence rate in the world [17]. Between the developed and developing nations of the world, *H. pylori* infection prevalence rate differs across the various regions [7]. Developed countries have been proven to experience less prevalence rate of *H. pylori* infection than the developing countries [17]. Researcher have observed that in a year about 0.5% of individual in the developed nations fall victim to *H. pylori* infection, but increases in the developing nations with the rates ranging from 3–10% [2, 19].

Among children in the developing countries, the prevalence rate of *H. pylori* infection ranges from below 10–80% [16], and from 1.8–65% among children in the developed countries [4]. It has been understood by epidemiological studies that some regions in the Eastern Asia and Latin American have recorded a prevalence rate of 80% among young individuals before 20 years, and places like UK, USA, or Australia records the prevalence rate of 40% within 30 to 40 years [7]. In the United States, observation has been made that *H. pylori* infection is rare among children lower than 10 years, but increases to 10% between the ages of 18 and 30 [7, 20]. In various nations like Canada, Netherlands, Mexico, Portugal, Asia, and Turkey according epidemiological studies have recorded *H. pylori* infection rate of 38, 32, 52, 84, 54–76%, and 82% respectively among children and adults [13, 21].

Data has revealed that individuals inhabiting industrialized countries have *H. pylori* infection rate ranging from 30–40% [13]. Also, among the non-Hispanic blacks and Hispanics, the infection of *H. pylori* is known to be common to individuals within any age group [2]. The African continent has been identified to have recorded a prevalence rate of 51% with regards to *H. pylori* infection [13]. Within the African countries like Ethiopia, Morocco, and Iran both children and adults according to studies have prevalence rate of 65, 75, and 54% respectively [13]. Organized data over the years have shown that *H. pylori* infections occurs within the early years of life, and increases with age [4]. By the first year of life in some developing countries, there is a prevalence rate of 20%, which increases to 50% by the age of 10 [2]. A research in Uganda showed that *H. pylori* infection varies with increasing age of 1–5 years, 6–10 years, and 11–15 years with 16.2, 27.2, and 36.71% as their respective prevalence rate [4]. The prevalence rate of *H. pylori* infection as revealed by studies in Nigeria, Indonesia, and Yemen were 89.7, 10.0, and 8.9% respectively [11].

4. Risk factors and mode of transmission

According to researched works, it has been understood that the increased *H. pylori* infection rate among the elderly is a direct mirror image of many early years of poor living conditions of the youngsters [2]. A study conducted in Bangladesh revealed lower infection rate of 4.9% among children living with family members below four, than those from the household having more than three members, corresponding to a rate of 19.4% [4]. Literature have established that socioeconomic status and childhood living conditions are highly associated with *H. pylori* infections [2]. Epidemiological studies have proven the fact that school going children, international adoptees, immigrant children are at high risk of developing *H. pylori* infection [4, 13]. It has also been identified that high risk children are those that usually swim in or drink from rivers, streams, ponds as well as consume raw vegetables. Generally, the major factors that put most children at risk of *H. pylori* infection includes poor personal and environmental hygiene, over-crowding areas, low socio-economic status, poor quality of drinking water, and eating of contaminated foods [7, 16, 22]. The level of urbanization also accounts for the variation of the prevalence rate of *H. pylori* infection among nations [11].

Microbiological strategies used in various studies have revealed that the micro-organism *H. pylori* can be found in contaminated environment and ground water, as well as in animals such as domestic cats and sheep worldwide [2, 7]. Irrespective of the fact that literature provides few information on the mode of transmission of the bacterium, epidemiological studies strongly support oral-oral, fecal-oral, and person-person, as well as zoonotic transmission [2, 4]. Infection routes limited to person-person transmission during the early stages of life could be possible from mothers, caretakers, nursery attendance, and family members to babies [3, 4]. Researched observations have been made that in the acquisition of *H. pylori* infections, genetic susceptibility is also possible [7, 13]. According to studies, exposure to diverse sources of *H. pylori* infection increases with the increasing ages of children [4, 23].

5. Pathosysiology

The stomach remains the primary colonization site for the bacterium *H. pylori* [6]. Though clear-cut understanding of the pathophysiology of *H. pylori* infection is not well known, it has been identified to cause both gastric and duodenal ulcers with multiple factors coming into play [2]. Literature has revealed the fact that 95% of duodenal ulcer and 70–80% of gastric ulcers are associated with *H. pylori* infec-tion [24]. There are four main strategic activities used by the bacterium *H. pylori* to facilitates its successful colonization, persistent infection, and disease pathogenesis [25]. The first of these basic but important strategies is its ability to survive within the stomach acidic condition, by producing urease to disrupt the acidic environ-ment, making it suitable and conducive to survive; secondly, its flagella facilitate movement to the epithelium cells of the stomach lining in order to attach itself, as well as to detect and live in the low pH region of the stomach; thirdly, it attaches the self to the host epithelial cells by adhesins preventing frequent displacement; and the fourth strategy is cell destruction or tissue damage, and this is done by the release of toxins called Cag A and Vac A [11, 25]. As the bacterium presents the self in the stomach lumen, it then localizes the self to the antrum and corpus for adaptation, so as to avoid the acidic condition of the stomach and to cause persistent infection [11]. Evidenced-based research works shows that cascades of destructive processes arise from the microorganism *H. pylori*'s interactions with the gastric epithelium of its host [26].

6. Clinical manifestation

Data have shown that about 30–35% of the individuals affected with *H. pylori* do not show any symptoms, especially among the young people [27]. Yet still it has been established that *H. pylori* infection tends to leave its victims with some form of gastric and entero-gastric manifestations [8]. According to studies, the combination of different factors like the host genetics, bacteria characteristics, and the environment account for the experience of various clinical manifestations by the affected individuals [13]. The manifestations that accompany *H. pylori* infection can either be associated with gastritis or Peptic ulcer disease [5]. Common signs and symptoms known to come along with this infection among the young people includes nausea, vomiting, gnawing or burning abdominal pain, intestinal bleeding, gastric reflex, occasional fever, poor appetite, bloating abdomen, frequent burping, tiredness and weakness, and weight loss [5, 23].

7. Complications

From literature review, it has been well proven that *H. pylori* infection comes along with both gastric and extra-gastric complications which are likely to be developed by the infected young person [28]. These various complications are due to late eradiation of the infection, and most of the times resulting from its asymptomatic nature at the early stage, as younger children hardly develop complications [11, 29]. The large range of gastric complications of *H. pylori* infection includes severe recurrent abdominal pain, gastric esophageal reflux (GER), gastric mucosa-associated lymphoid tissue lymphoma (MALT), Peptic ulcer disease, gastric adenocarcinoma, chronic gastritis, and others [4]. Also, some extra-gastric conditions that may be present in the delay eradication of the infection among the young people includes iron deficiency anemia, chronic idiopathic thrombocytopenic purpura, growth retardation, diabetes mellitus, coronary heart disease, normal tension glaucoma and others [9, 28].

Studies reveal that more than 50% of the children in Europe affected with *H. pylori* experience retarded growth [24]. Different literatures have presented with the fact that young people who have acquired *H. pylori* infection have 1–2% life time risk of developing stomach cancer, whiles 60–70% are likely to develop gastric mucosa-associated lymphoid tissue lymphoma (MALT) [19, 24, 29, 30]. Complications like gastric cancer resulting from *H. pylori* infection has been proven to be a significant health problem in the world, as identified to be the third most major cause of cancer-related mortality of 723,100 in the year 2012 [11].

8. Diagnostic investigations

Scientists have done their possible best to make available various scientific means to help diagnose individuals who have been infected with *H. pylori* [6]. Although *H. pylori* infection can be acquired globally, regular test for the presence of *H. pylori* among individuals are not recommended due to the fact that most patients do not develop significant gastro duodenal disease [2]. The European Helicobacter Study Group recommended that diagnostic investigation should be done for children with family history of Peptic ulcer disease, and chronic abdominal pain [2]. Testing and eradication therapy is only requested for infected individuals who are suspected of developing Peptic ulcer disease so as to reduce the rate of antibiotic resistance [13]. According to literature, the various diagnostic investigations have been categorized into invasive or endoscopic test and non-invasive or non-endoscopic test [2, 6].

Non-invasive scientific methods include Urea breath test with a sensitivity rate of 90–96% and specificity rate of 88–98%, Antibody test has sensitivity rate of 88–94% and specificity rate of 74–88% [2, 12], and Fecal Antigen test which also has sensitivity rate of 91–96% and specificity rate of 95–96% [31]. Invasive diagnostic test is also made up of histology, and it has a sensitivity rate of 93–96% and specificity rate of 98–99%, Culture has a sensitivity rate of 80–98% and specificity rate of 100%, Rapid Urea test has a sensitivity rate of 88–95% and specificity rate of 95–100%, as well as Polymerase Chain reaction which has a sensitivity rate above 95% and specificity rate also above 95% [2]. As revealed by studies, two or more tests are very much required to accurately establish the present of the bacterium *H. pylori* [3, 22]. Also, non-invasive methods are more reliable among the young people before and after treatment, whereas the invasive ones are difficult to perform among younger children [3, 5, 31, 32].

9. Management

The management of the infection *H. pylori* is based on three main criteria including destroying the micro bacterium *H. pylori*, treating the ulcer present either in the stomach or duodenum, and to prevent the recurrent of the infection which can be possible after 7 to 14 days of treatment [33]. Studies have shown that the only effective management strategy to reduce *H. pylori* associated with gastric cancer and extra-gastric complication is the eradication regimen [11]. In 70–95% of the cases, eradication of the microorganism is successful whereas 50–80% of the cases progress into cancers [33]. The triple therapies have been reported to have sufficient therapeutic rate of 85–90% [34, 35]. Antibiotics such as Amoxicillin, Clarithromycin, Metronidazole, Tetracycline, or Tinidazole can be used to kill the bacterium [33]. Dexlansoprazole, Esomeprazole, Lansoprazole, or Omeprazole can be used to decrease the secretion of gastric acid within the stomach by blocking its production source [33]. Cimetidine, Famotidine, Nizatidine, or Ranitidine is usually used to inhibit histamine that mediate the production of the gastric acidic content that is likely to erode the wall lining of the stomach [33]. Among individuals with *H. pylori* infection, surgery as treatment is not an option, but can be recommended only for victims that are developing severe complications like the malignancies [34].

It has been identified that the first-line eradication management for standard triple therapy must be Amoxicillin, Clarithromycin, and Proton-pump inhibit (PPI) for a time period of 14 days [34, 36]. PPI, Metronidazole, Amoxicillin, and Clarithromycin have been proven to have eradication efficiency rate of 84.3% [11]. In order to confirm the complete eradication of *H. pylori* infection, treated patients must be tested again even after management [13]. Higher weight-based doses of Proton-pump inhibitor (PPI) management regimen are what young children need as against the adolescents and the elderly, and it has also been proved to be very efficient in dealing with the eradication of the infection [13]. However, the test-and-treat management strategy is less recommended for young patients below the age of 14 years [36]. Studies have shown that washing of hands thoroughly and frequently, drinking of safe water, as well as eating well prepared foods can help prevent the infection of *H. pylori* among the youngsters [5]. Recently, studies have recommended the addition of iron therapy in the management and establishment of *H. pylori* infection eradication [10]. In the eradication therapy strategy, sequential therapy has been proven to command positive results of more than 90% efficiency [10]. The duration of the eradication therapy is also very much important, and research studies as well as commendation from the European and United States indicates that 14 days of sequential treatment is the most potent among the durations 7,10, or 14 days [37].

10. Rate of antibiotics resistance

There are few numbers of antibiotics used in the treatment of *H. pylori* infection among children [36]. The increase rate of antibiotic resistance to the management of *H. pylori* infection has become obvious [38]. Therefore, recommendations have been made that drug susceptibility test is to be conducted before treatment so as to identify the corresponding regimen needed for accurate management [3]. A study conducted in Cameroon in the year 2019 revealed that Amoxicillin and Metronidazole have the highest resistance rate of 97.14% and 97.85% respectively, and so recommendation was made that they should be avoided as components of the triple therapy in the eradication of *H. pylori* infection especially among the young people [38]. In countries like Nepal and Bangladesh, Metronidazole resistance rate recorded by studies were 88 and 84% respectively [11]. Another study conducted in Vietnam showed that Clarithromycin, Levofloxacin, and Tetracycline have the resistance rate of 34.1, 29.7, and 17.9% respectively [39]. Common treatment strategies for *H. pylori* eradication have been observed to have a failure rate of 20% [37].

The resistance rate of Clarithromycin increased from 13% in the year 2006 to 21% by the year 2016 [39]. Countries such as China, Turkey, Japan and Italy, and Sweden and Taiwan have recorded Clarithromycin resistance rate of 50, 40, 30, and 15% respectively [10]. A study conducted among isolates revealed a multiple drug resistance pattern of 42.57% double therapy, 15.71% triple therapy, and 5.71% quadruple therapy [38]. There is a high antibiotic resistance rate in *H. pylori* infection than in other bacteria, due to the increase misuse and overuse of antibiotics for the treatment of other infections in most developing nations [11]. Some contributing factors such as inability to responding to treatment, and gastric suppressant inadequacy results in antibiotic resistance among young people [34]. Due to the great impact of the resistance in the treatment of *H. pylori*, World Health Organization (WHO) in the year 2017 identified it as part of the common cause of community-acquired infection [11]. It has been recommended that second line therapy be included in the eradication of *H. pylori* since the first line therapy has been observed to have about 20% rate of failure [37].

11. Conclusion

Numerous factors might play different roles in the development of Peptic ulcer disease, but one significant biological factor that has been associated with the occurrence of this global gastrointestinal health problem is the *H. pylori*. Poor socio-economic status, poor personal and environmental hygiene, drinking contaminated water, eating contaminated food, and overcrowded arears have been identified to make school going children more prone to developing *H. pylori* infection at the early stages of life. *H. pylori* infection is associated with gastritis, and gastric ulcers. Therefore, early detection and effective treatment of the infection is needed to well establish its eradication and further prevent any clinical complications likely to develop in the later years of life. In the aspect of prevalence rate, complications, rare occurrence of malignancies, age-specific problems with diagnostic test and drugs, as well as for increased rate of antibiotic resistant, children differ from the elderly in terms of *H. pylori* infection. Therefore, some recommendations for the elderly may not be relevant to the youngsters.

Acknowledgements

Extending sincere gratitude to all authors and publishers of the books and articles used as reference in this research work. Good wishes to all who will find this researched work useful in their various field of study. Many appreciations and gratitude to the sponsors and funders of this researched work. Thank you.

Author details

Sampson Weytey
Valley View University, Accra, Ghana

*Address all correspondence to: sampsonweytey@gmail.com

IntechOpen

References

[1] Uyanikoghi A, Danaliogulu A, Akuz F, Pinarbasi B, Gulluoglu M, Kapoan Y, et al. In: Chai J, editor. The Etiological Factors of Duodenal and Gastric Ulcers Peptic Ulcer Disease. Apr 2011;**23**(2):99-103. Available from: https://www.intechopen.com

[2] Tsang T, Shresth MP. Helico bacter pylori Infection in Peptic Ulcer Disease. Peptic Ulcer Disease. Nov, 2011;(3). Rijeka, Jianyan Chai: Intechopen; Available from: https://doi.org/10.5772/24889

[3] Okuda M, Lin Y, Kikuchi S. *Helicobacter pylori* infection in children and adolescent. In: Kamiya S, Backert S, editors. *Helicobacter pylori* in Human Disease. Advanced in Experimental Medicine and Biology. Vol. 1149. Cham: Springer; 2019. https://doi.org/10.1007/554_2019-361

[4] Aitala P, Mutyaba M, Okeny S, Kasule NM, Kasule R, Ssedyabane F, et al. Prevalence and risk factors of *Helicobacter pylori* infection among children aged 1-15 years at Holy Innocents Children Hospital, Mbaraba, South Western Uganda. Journal of Tropical Medicine. 2019: Vol. p 6. Article ID 9303072, 10.1155/2019/9303072

[5] Denham MJ. Helico bacter pylori. Gastroenterology. Nemours Children's Health. 2021. Reviewed article. Available from: https://www.kidshealth.org/en/parents /h-pylori.html on the 10th September, 2021.

[6] Salles N. *Helicobacter pylori* infection in elderly patients. In: Chai J, editor. Peptic Ulcer Disease. Rijeka, JianyanCha: Intechopen; Nov 2011;(14). https://www.intechopen.com

[7] Parra-cid T, Fernandez CM, Gisbert PJ. Helicobacter pylori and peptic ulcer-role of reactive oxygen species and apoptosis. In: Chai J, editor. Peptic Ulcer Disease. Nov, 2011;(9). Rijeka: JianyanChai; https://www.intechopen.com

[8] Nordestgaard MA, Spiegelhauer RM, Frandsen HT, Gren C, Stauning AT, Andersen PL. Open access-review chapter. In: Clinical Manifestation of Epsilon Proteobacteria (*Helicobacter pylori*). 2018;(2). DOI: https://doi:5772/intechopen.8033

[9] Pacifico L, Osborn FJ, Tromba V, Bascetta S, Romaggioli S, Chiesa C. Helicobacter pylori and extra-gastric disorder in children: A critical update. World Journal of Grastroenterology. 2014;**20**(6):1379-1401. DOI: https://doi:10.3748./wjg.v20.i 6.1379

[10] Diaconu S, Predesco A, Moldoveanu A, Pop CS, Fierbinteanu-Braticevici C. Helicobacter pylori infection: Old and new. Journal of Medicine and Life. 2017;**10**(20):112-117 https://www.ncbi.nlm.nih.gov/pmc/articles/PMC5467250/#_Hn_sectitle

[11] Ansari S, Yamaoka Y. Current understanding and management of Helicobacter pylori infection: An update appraisal Version 1. F1000Res Faculty Rev-721. 2018;7:F1000. DOI: 10.12688/f1000research.14149.1

[12] Dunn BE, Coher H, Blaser MJ.Helico bacter pylori. Clinical Microbiology Reviews. 2021. Vol 10, Number 4, pages 720-741. Pub Med: 9336670. Available from: https://doi.org/10.1128/CMR.10.4.720 on the 6th September, 2021.

[13] Korotkaya Y, Shores D. Helicobacter pylori in pediatric patients. Pediatrics in Review. November 2020;**41**(11): 585-592. https://doi.org/10.1542/pir.2019-0048

[14] Kalach N, Bontems P, Josette R. Helicobacter pylori infection in children. 2017;**22**(S1):e1241. Available on https://doi.org/10.1111/hel.12414

[15] Abadi ATB. Strategies used by *Helicobacter pylori* to establish persistence infection. World Journal of Gastroenterology. 28 Apr 2017;**28**(16): 2870-2882. https://doi:10.3748/wjg.v23. i16.2870. PMID:28522905; PMCID: PMC5413782

[16] Kyle AB, Steensma PD, Shampo AM. Barry James Marshall-Discovery of Helicobacter pylori as a cause of peptic ulcer. Stamp Vignette on Medical Science. 2016;**91**(5):E67-E68. https:// doi.org/10.1016/j.May06.2016.01.025

[17] Samily AM, Morshed MA. An update of labouratory diagnosis of Helicobacter pylori in the Kingdom of Saudi Arabia. Journal of Intectious Dev Ctries. 2015;**9**(8):806-814. https:// doi:10.355/jidc.542

[18] Silva MIG, Florencode Sousa F. Gastric ulceretiology. Peptic Ulcer Disease. Rijeka: Jianyan Chai Intechopen; Nov, 2011;**2011**(1). https:// doi.org/10.5772/20796.

[19] Ankouane F, Noah ND, Enyime NF, Ndjolle MC, Djapa NR, Nonga NB, Njoya O, Ndam NCL. Helicobacter pylori and precancerous conditions of the stomach: The frequency of infection in a cross-sectional study of 79 consecutive patients with chronic antral gastritis in Yaounde, Cameroon. The Pan African Medical Journal. 2015; **20**:52. https://doi:10.11604/Pamj.2015. 20:52.5887

[20] Park SJ, Jun SJ, Seo JH, Youn HS, Rhee HK. Changing prevalence of Helicobacter pylori infection in children and adolescent. Clinical and Experimental Pediatric. 2021;**64**(1):21-25. https://doi. org/10.3345/cep.2019.01543

[21] Soltan J, Amirzadeh J, Nahedi S, Shahsavari S. Prevalence of helicobacter pylori in children; a population-based cross-sectional study in West Iran. Iranian Journal of Pediatrics. 2013;**23**(1): 13-18. PMCID: PMC354986

[22] Falck S. Helicobacter pylori infection. Healthline Media. 2019. Update on March 26, 2019. Available from: https://www. healthline.com/health/helicobacter pylori#complications on the 4th September, 2021.

[23] Cochran JW. Pepticulcer disease in children. MSD Manual Consumer Version. Reviewed on August 2021. 2021. Available from https://www. msdmanuals.com/home/children-s- health/issues/digestive disorders-in- children/peptic-ulcer-in children on the 9th September, 2021.

[24] Akcam M, Aslan N. *Helicobacter pylori* related health problems in children. Iran Journal of Public Health. 2015;**44**(6):877-878. PMCID:4524316 PMID:26258104

[25] Ka, CY, Sheu BS, Wu JJ. *Helicobacter pylori* infection: An overview of bacterial virulence factors and pathogenesis. Biomedical Journal. 2016;**39**(1):14-23. ISSN 2319-4170. https://www.sciencedirect.com/science/ article/pii/S2319417016000160

[26] Gonciarz W, Krupa A, Hinc K, Obuchowaski M, Moran AP, Gajewski A, Chmiela M. The effects of Helicobacter pylori infection and different Helicobacter pylori components on the proliferation and apoptosis of gastric epithelial cells and fibroblast. PLoS ONE. 2019;**14**(8): e0220636. https://doi:10.1371/journal. pone.0220636

[27] Senbanjo OI, Oshikoya AK, Njokanma FO. Helicobacter pylori associated with breastfeeding, nutritional status, and recurrent abdominal pain in healthy Nigerian children. Journal of Infection in Developing Countries. 2014;**8**(4): 448-453. https://doi:10.3855/jide.3196

[28] Ali AM, Elkhabit WF. Potential complication of Helicobacter pylori infection in children of non-urban

community. Archives of Pediatric Infectious Diseases.2015;**3**(2): e23512. https://doi:10.5812/pedinfect.23510

[29] Gulcan M, Ozen A, Karatep OH, Vitrinel A. Impact of Helicobacter pylori on growth: Is the infection or the mucosal disease related to growth impairment? Digestive Diseases and Sciences. 2010;**55**: 2878-2886. https://doi.rog/10.1007/S10620-009-1091-Y

[30] Hestvik T, Tylleskar T, Kaddu-Mulindwa DH, Tumwine KJ. Helicobacter pylori in apparently healthy children aged 0-12 years in Urban Kampala, Uganda: A community-based cross-sectional survey. BMC Gastroenterology. 2010;**10**:62. https://doi.org/10.1186/1471-230X-10-62

[31] Gold DB, Gilger AM, Czinn JS. New diagnostic strategies for the detection of *Helicobacter pylori* infection in pediatric patients. Gastroenterología y Hepatología. 2014;**12**(Suppl 7):1-19

[32] Khatri M. What is *Helicobacter pylori*? Medically Reviewed on 7th December, 2020. 10th September, 2021. Available from: https://www.webmd.com/diagestive-disorders/h-pylori-helicobacter-pylori

[33] Santacroce L. Helicobacter pylori infection and management. Medscape Medical News. 5 September 2021. Available from: https://emedicine.medscape.com/article/176938-treatment

[34] Nestegar O, Johnsen KM, Sorbye SW, Halvorsen FA, Tonnessen T, Paulssen EJ, et al. Helicobacter pylori infected patients 15 years after successful eradication. PLoS ONE. 2020;**15**(9):e0238944. DOI: https://doi:10.1371/journal.pone.0238944

[35] Li J, Deng J, Wang Z, Li H, Wan C. Antibiotic resistance of *Helicobacter pylori* strains isolated from pediatric patients in southwest China. ORIGINAL RESEARCH article. Frontiers in Microbiology. 2021;**11**: 621791. 26 January 2021 | https://doi.org/10.3389/fmicb.2020.621791

[36] Jemilohun CA, Otegbayo JA. Helicobacter pylori infection: Past, present, and future. Original article. The Pan African Medical Journal. 2016;**23**:Article 216. 10.1164. pamj. 23.216.8852. https://www.panafrican-med-journal.com/content/article/23/216/full

[37] Kouitcheu Mabeku LB, Eyoum Bille B, Tepap Zemnou C, et al. Broad spectrum resistance in Helicobacter pylori isolated from gastric biopsies of patients with dyspepsia in Cameroon and efflux-mediated multiresistance detection in MDR isolates. BMC Infectious Diseases. 2019;**19**:880. https://doi.org/10.1186/s12879-019-4536-8

[38] Khien VV, Thang MD, Hai MT, Duat NQ, Khanh PH, Ha DT, et al. Management of antibiotic-resistant Helicobacter pylori infection: Perspectives from Vietnam. Gut Liver. Sep 2019;**13**(5):483-497. Published online 2019 Apr 23. DOI: 10.5009/gnl18137. PMCID: PMC674379. PMID: 31009957

[39] Savoldi A,Carrara E,Graham DY, Conti M, Tacconelli E. Prevalence of Antibiotic Resistance in Helicobacter pylori: A systematic Review and Metaanalysis inWorld Health Organization Regions. Gastroenterology. Nov 2018;**155**(5):1372-1382.e17. Available from: https://doi.org/10.1053/j.gastro.2018.07.007. Epub 2018Jul7. PMID: 29990487; PMCID: PMC6905086

Chapter 3

Peptic Ulcer Disease

Carlos A. Casalnuovo, Pedro A. Brégoli,
Cesar J. Valdivieso Duarte and Carlos A. Vera Cedeño

Abstract

Peptic ulcer disease, including duodenal and gastric ulcers, is associated with potentially life-threatening complications, including bleeding, perforation, and gastric outlet obstruction. Stomach lesions are located preferentially along the small curvature in the transition zone between the body and the antrum; in the duodenum those lesions are located in the duodenal bulb, where posterior lesions are usually associated with hemorrhage and the anterior ones with perforation. Peptic ulcer disease affects approximately 5–10% of the population worldwide and represents an important cost for public health. Peptic ulcers pathogenesis is complex and involves multifactorial processes, which basically occurs by an imbalance between aggressive and defensive factors of the gastric mucosa. Gastric mucosa is continuously exposed to harmful substances and factors, whether endogenous (acid secretion, peptic activity, and biliary secretion) or exogenous (Helicobacter pylori infection, alcohol abuse, smoking habit, and nonsteroidal anti-inflammatory drugs (NSAIDs)) and stressful life habits.

Keywords: peptic ulcer disease, bleeding, perforation, gastric outlet obstruction, gastric ulcer complications

1. Introduction

Peptic ulcer disease (PUD) is common with a lifetime prevalence in the general population of 5–10% and an incidence of 0.1–0.3% per year. Peptic ulceration occurs due to acid peptic damage to the gastroduodenal mucosa, resulting in mucosal erosion that exposes the underlying tissues to the digestive action of gastroduodenal secretions. This pathology was traditionally related to a hypersecretory acid environment, dietary factors, and stress. However, the increasing incidence of the Helicobacter pylori infection, the extensive use of NSAIDs, and the increase in alcohol and smoking abuse have changed the epidemiology of this disease. Despite a sharp reduction in incidence and rates of hospital admission and mortality over the past 30 years, complications are still encountered in 10–20% of these patients. Complications of peptic ulcer disease include perforation and bleeding, and improvement in medical management has made obstruction from chronic fibrotic disease a rare event [1].

2. Bleeding

Bleeding is a common complication and the leading cause of death from peptic ulcer. Requiring endoscopic therapy in the onset of bleeding, rebleeding and multiple comorbidities are predictive of mortality. Treatment often requires the participation of a multidisciplinary team.

2.1 Definition

Upper gastrointestinal bleedings (UGBs) are those originating proximal to Treitz angle, including diseases of the esophagus, stomach, duodenum, and those generating haemobilia, such as tumors or trauma of the liver, bile duct, and pancreas. Approximately 20% of peptic ulcers have an episode of bleeding, and 25–30% of them repeat it.

2.2 Pathophysiology

The wall of the stomach has a complex irrigation. By eroding the wall, peptic ulcers may injure a large vessel causing bleeding; once it starts, gastric acid becomes more harmful because a pH of 6 or below diminishes platelet aggregation and clots get unstable. In the duodenum, irrigation comes from the gastroduodenal and pancreaticoduodenal arteries, which are larger in the posterior wall, and that's why the majority of hemorrhage complications are related to posterior wall duodenal ulcers. Loss of intravascular volume leads to shock, the severity of which is determined primarily by the amount, speed, and body's ability to compensate blood lost. Hypovolemia causes a reduction in tissue perfusion. The first compensation phenomena are the release of catecholamines that generate vasoconstriction.

2.3 Clinical presentation

The initial management is essential. Based on the grade of hypovolemia, the patient may be hemodynamically compensated or need an urgent transfusion. Treatment depends on patient's general condition after bleeding onset. Clinical presentation may be oligosymptomatic, with or without history of PUD symptoms, and without rebleeding it would whether go unnoticed or be diagnosed in a follow-up check, usually by anemia; it would also be presented as a complication in the evolution of a previously diagnosticated peptic ulcer. Almost 30% of ulcers begin their clinical manifestations with bleeding.

Bleeding can also be classified based on the percentage of blood lost, into:

MILD, if the loss is less than 10% of the total blood volume.

MODERATE, when it is 10 to 20%.

SEVERE, with a loss of more than 20% of the total blood volume.

There is also another classification according to the volume lost and the consequent management (**Table 1**).

Taking the history of the patient should identify those patients with systemic diseases that may predispose or promote bleeding such as gastric or duodenal

	ml	Blood volume (%)	Treatment
I	<750	<15	Fluids
II	750–1500	15–30	Fluids
III	1500–2000	30–40	Fluids + blood
IV	>2000	>40	Fluids + blood

Table 1.
Hypovolemic classification.

pathology, liver disease that predisposes to coagulopathies, portal hypertension, stress situations, and use of NSAIDs or anticoagulants.

2.3.1 Signs and symptoms

Hematemesis is usually absent in mild bleeding, while melena (tarry stools) is evident with 50–100 ml of blood. The presence or absence of hematochezia depends on the bleeding rate and the speed of bowel transit. The paleness of the skin and mucous membranes depends on the degree of anemia, while orthostatism is one of the first symptoms of hypovolemia.

2.4 Diagnosis

In cases with doubts, a nasogastric tube may show traces of blood or active bleeding, with a 10% of false-negatives.

2.4.1 Physical examination

As bleeding progresses, tachycardia, arterial hypotension, tachypnea, oliguria, poor peripheral perfusion, Glasgow deterioration, and shock appear. Digital rectal exam can evaluate rectal content and differentiate between melena and red blood.

2.4.2 Laboratory

Hematocrit: In acute bleeding and the first hours, it is practically not modified then it is more useful for the replacement of the blood volume lost and control for eventually rebleeding scenario. Anemia without signs of hypovolemia suggests slow bleeding (chronic anemia). In UGB, the elevation of urea in the blood is very common, without being part of diagnostic criteria.

2.4.3 Endoscopy

It is the main diagnostic procedure with an efficiency of 80 to 90%. It has three goals: to make a diagnosis, to stop bleeding, and to assess the risk of rebleeding. Endoscopy should not be deferred. It evaluates:

1. Topographic diagnosis. Location of the bleeding lesion (esophagus, stomach, or duodenum) and other possible lesions. Endoscopy is essential due to the possibility of treatment, since bleeding endoscopic treatment may avoid gastrotomies or duodenotomies.

2. Etiological diagnosis. Both tactics and opportunity change depending on the cause and pace of bleeding.

3. Evaluation of the "Type of Bleeding". Forrest et al. [2] (**Table 2**) described the characteristics of bleeding lesions, to unify diagnostic and prognostic criteria.

4. Application of a therapeutic procedure (**Figures 1–4**).

Other options of exceptional need, given the persistence of bleeding without endoscopic findings, are:

Forrest classification		Rebleeding (%)
I. Active bleeding	Ia. Spurting hemorrhage (**Figure 1**)	90–100
	Ib. Oozing hemorrhage (**Figure 2**)	80–85
II. Signs of recent bleeding	IIa. Non-bleeding visible vessel (**Figure 3**)	40–45
	IIb. Adherent clot on lesion (**Figure 4**)	20–30
	IIc. Hematin-covered lesion	5
III. Lesion without bleeding		<3

Table 2.
Forrest classification.

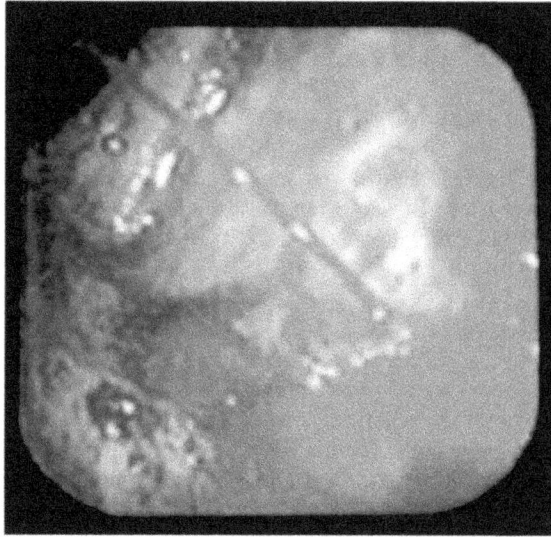

Figure 1.
Spurting hemorrhage.

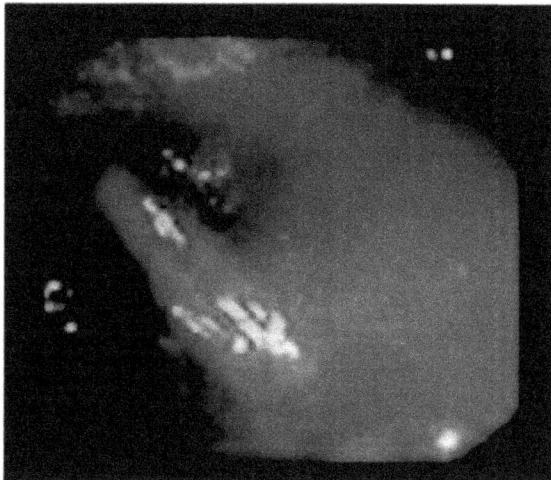

Figure 2.
Oozing hemorrhage.

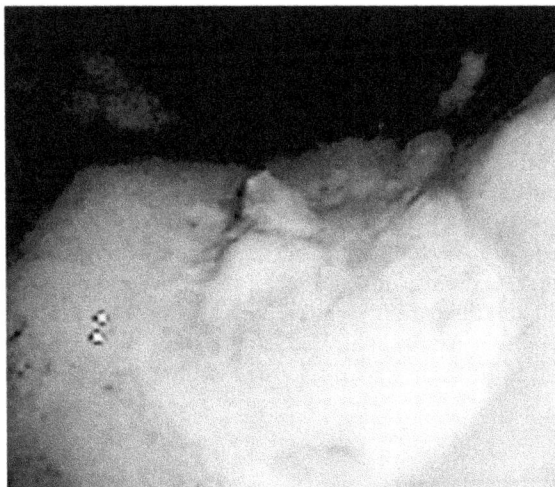

Figure 3.
Non-bleeding visible vessel.

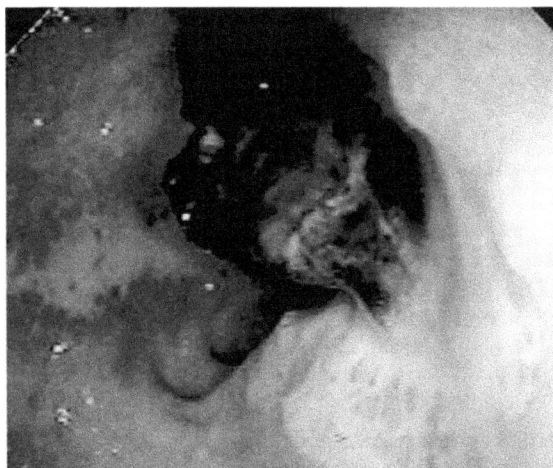

Figure 4.
Adherent clot on lesion.

2.4.4 Selective arteriography

Sensitivity depends on the bleeding extent and the operator. Lesions such as tumors or vascular malformations can be detected even if they are not bleeding at the time of the study. Arteriography could also be therapeutic by the possibility of eventual embolization, making this technique analog to endoscopy (diagnostic and therapeutic). Topographically locates the bleeding area if there is a loss greater than 0.5 cc/minute.

2.4.5 99mTc-labeled red cell scintigraphy

A technetium Tc 99m-labeled red cell scan is another diagnostic resource with specific indications and may be helpful in localizing the source of bleeding, although with brisk bleeding the time required for the scan is problematic and urgent surgical intervention may be more expeditious. Topographically locates the bleeding area if there is a loss greater than 0.2 cc/minute.

2.5 Natural evolution

It is estimated that more than 70% of UGB by peptic ulcer respond to medical treatment. Adding endoscopic to medical treatments, the bleeding control reach 90%. Rebleeding is a proven prognostic factor. With an effective endoscopic procedure, it is only seen in 10% of those under 60 years old and in 15–20% of those over 60 years. The worst scenario of rebleeding is when the endoscopic treatments are already exhausted and the patient remains with hypovolemia, and increasingly in worse conditions which usually contraindicates getting the patient to the operation room. Between 5 and 10%, they are discharged without etiological diagnosis.

2.6 Treatment

2.6.1 Medical treatment

After initial evaluation of the patient, fluid resuscitation may be achieved by canalizing two peripheral veins with 14 Fr catheters. Due to persistence of hypovolemia (hypotension) without response to fluid resuscitation, blood transfusion is mandatory. Hypovolemic shock would require the placement of a central venous catheter that measures venous pressure, or Swan-Ganz catheter placement to measure the pressure in the pulmonary artery when the shock is severe. Simultaneously and according to severity, a mechanical ventilation is evaluated in order to achieve integral life support management.

Catheterization of the bladder is to control urine output. A nasogastric tube is useful if there is Glasgow deterioration, to prevent regurgitation of gastric contents to the airway. It can also evaluate bleeding; aspiration favors an eventual endoscopy.

A gastric pH > 6 is ideal to decrease the risk of rebleeding. In 95% of cases, it is achieved with proton pump inhibitors (PPIs) in intravenous doses of 40–80 mg/day.

2.6.2 Endoscopic treatment

Until the mid-80s, endoscopy was only diagnostic. Nowadays, it is very common to attempt for endoscopic hemostasia before indicating surgical treatment.

The most accepted technique is the adrenaline or epinephrine 1:10,000 injection, and better results would be obtained if sclerosing agents such as ethanolamine oleate, human thrombin, or cauterization are added. Other methods such as bipolar electrocautery (**Figure 5**), laser (**Figures 6** and 7), elastic bands, or hemo-clips are effective but require more training and specific equipment. Currently, endoscopic treatments are effective in more than 90% of cases.

Hemostasis in lesions with pulsatile bleeding have more than a 50% chance of rebleeding, but it also facilitates hemodynamic stabilization until surgical intervention. In those with a visible vessel without active bleeding, the incidence of rebleeding is 40–50%, while lesions with a clot adhered rebleeding rate is estimated around 20–30%, so a second endoscopic treatment is suggested at 48 h.

2.7 Rebleeding

It is defined as a new episode of hematemesis and/or melena, associated with signs of hypovolemia or anemia. This must be confirmed by endoscopy. The risk

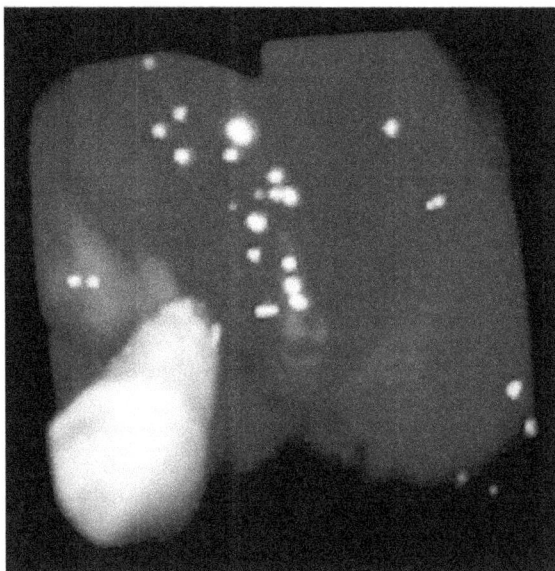

Figure 5.
Rebleeding.

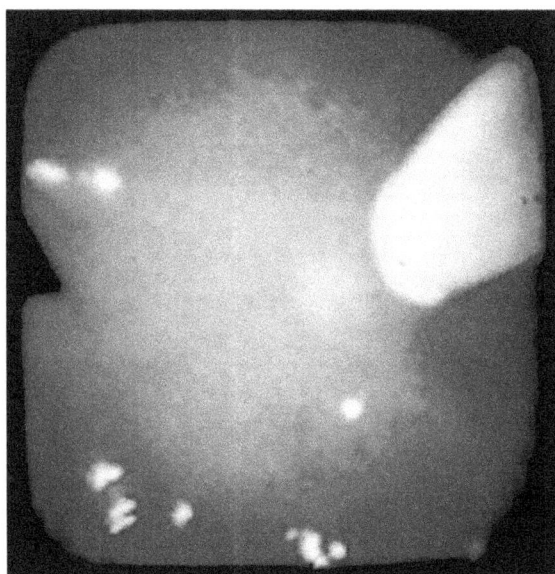

Figure 6.
Endoscopic treatment.

of rebleeding depends on several factors, such as, massive UGB, persistence of hemodynamic instability, delay endoscopic treatment, larger size of the ulcer, those having a visible vessel or a clot attached, even without active bleeding and posterior duodenal ulcers.

After endoscopic treatment, administration of proton pump inhibitors decreases rebleeding risk.

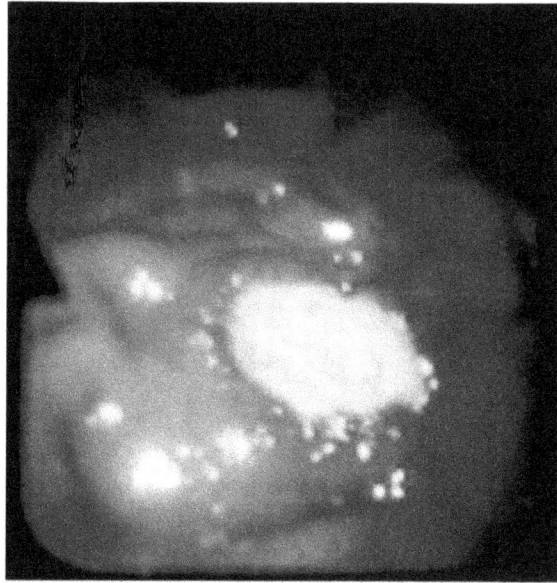

Figure 7.
Endoscopic electrocoagulation of an active bleeding.

2.8 Surgical treatment

Modern medical and endoscopic treatments have decreased the frequency of operations for upper gastrointestinal bleeding.

Surgical indication:

The criteria or guides that stand out are:

1. Magnitude of bleeding

   Hypovolemic shock has a "period of reversibility," so if hemodynamic stability is not achieved, an operation should be chosen.

   According to this criterion, surgery is indicated when bleeding requires more than five blood units in the first 24 h.

2. Persistence of bleeding

   Between 5 and 10% of patients with UGB keep bleeding once the initial hypovolemia is controlled and even after medical and endoscopic treatments.

   With these criteria, the operation is indicated when there is a daily requirement of two blood units, for 4 days or more.

3. Rebleeding

   It occurs between 10 and 30% of the hemorrhages already treated. It is recommended that patients at high risk of rebleeding should have a new evaluation in the following 2 or 3 days. In the face of new bleeding, the surgical indication

is urgent, because treatment alternatives are exhausted, the failure of a new endoscopic procedure is very high, and the patient deteriorates rapidly.
Surgical tactics:
The main objectives of the operation are:

1. Control of bleeding

2. The cure of ulcerative disease, if feasible, but is not the main objective. Maintaining postoperative PPI therapy is mandatory.

In the plan matters patient general condition, the history of the PUD, its location, the operative risk, and the experience of the surgical team.

2.8.1 Gastric ulcer (GU)

Surgeons have two options:

1. Hemostatic suture

   It is the first option because of its simplicity and results and is indicated also in patients who had not received right medical treatment. The hemostatic suture consists of making deep suture throughout the extension of the ulcer, with nonabsorbable material or very slow absorption and using semicircular and strong needles, due to sclerosis of the peri-ulcerous tissue.

2. Gastrectomy

   It is feasible in compensated patients. As the most frequent gastric ulcers are in the middle and distal thirds, the most used operations are antrectomies and hemigastrectomies, trying to avoid subtotal resections. The need for a total gastrectomy for PUD is exceptional. When the procedure does not include resection of the ulcer, biopsies should be taken before hemostasia, for the chance of having a bleeding carcinoma.

2.8.2 Duodenal ulcer (DU)

There are several options.

1. Hemostatic suture (**Figure 8**): currently, it is the most used technique in non-compensated and compensated patients. Because PPIs and H. pylori eradication cure more than 90% of DU, hemostatic suture and medical treatment from the immediate postoperative period have goods results and lowers risks. The technique of hemostasia is like in GU, adding an important difference in posterior wall ulcers due to their proximity to the bile duct. Another complementary option is the external ligation of the vessel that irrigates the anatomic portion where the ulcer is located.

2. Hemostasia and vagotomy with gastric drainage: in compensated patients and with chronic ulcer disease, adding a vagotomy with drainage to the hemostatic suture is a physio-pathologically correct criterion, but less used today. The reduction in acid secretion achieved with vagotomy is lower or the same in some cases as with proton pump inhibitors.

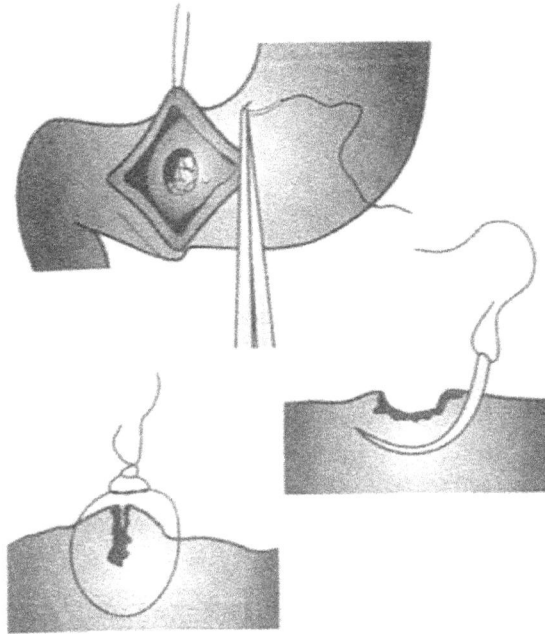

Figure 8.
Longitudinally pyloro-duodenotomy and posterior defect transversal closure (pyloroplasty).

2.9 Mortality

Mortality in patients admitted to hospital with UGB ranges between 5 and 10%, while in intensive care units, when there is bleeding as a complication of another serious disease, it can exceed 25%.

3. Perforated peptic ulcers

Perforations begin penetrating the layers of the viscera until they open freely in the peritoneum or are blocked by neighboring tissues or organs. They occur between 2 and 10% of patients with PU.

Perforation is a frequent cause of acute abdomen. The perforation causes the leak of chlorohydric acid in to the peritoneum, constituting over time in to septic shock.

3.1 Diagnosis

3.1.1 History

In 70% of those perforated, there is a history of ulcerative disease or a known diagnosis of GU or DU. The remaining 30% is divided between those who are perforated without previous symptoms and those who present symptoms of PU a few weeks before perforation. The pain of the perforation is very intense, with an abrupt beginning and mid-abdominal predominance. Then it becomes continuous and spreads to the rest of the abdomen with propagation to the chest and shoulders. The intensity of the pain causes sweating, paleness, and superficial breathing. Peritoneal irritation causes an antalgic position to be adopted with the thighs flexed over the abdomen.

With time, fever, arterial hypotension, ileus, and oliguria are added, and eventually if not treated achieving systemic failure.

3.1.2 Physical examination

Paleness of the skin and mucous membranes, tachycardia, and hypotension are common findings. When peritonitis is already installed, the patient is still and does not try to move. In the palpation of the abdomen, there is muscle contracture, (rigid abdomen) defense, and pain to decompression (Blumberg sign). The disappearance of hepatic dullness to percussion is a classical semiological maneuver (Jobert's sign), which must be followed by radiological studies. It means the interposition of air between the liver and the abdominal wall (Popper's sign).

Perforated ulcers are a constant surgical pathology at pace with advances in the medical treatment of peptic ulcer disease.

In 1987, Boey and Wong [3] scientifically analyzed several risk factors to conclude that mortality significantly increased

a. when there was preoperative shock;

b. when there were serious associated diseases; and

c. when treatment was started more than 24 h after perforation (most studies had used a 12-h parameter). Diffuse peritoneal contamination aged over 60 years and less than 3 months of ulcerative history had no value as isolated factors, but when they were associated with others.

The analysis of 613 perforations in Hong Kong recorded only 22.2% with one or more of the three main risk factors, which influenced the low overall mortality of 4.7%.

In 1989, we applied several risk factors to a retrospective series of 105 perforated at the "Hospital de Clinicas" [4]. Ninety-two percent had one or more of the following factors: (a) onset time of more than 12 h; (b) concomitance of associated serious diseases; (c) over 60 years of age, which led to a mortality of 26.7%. The first factor is related to the delay in treatment (58.1% had more than 12 h of perforation). Sometimes, the blame lays with the patient and their family members, but other times it is due to failures of primary medical care.

In our series, 33.3% were over the age of 60 years and 28.6% received corticosteroids or NSAID, figures similar to those of Watkins et al. [5].

When we evaluated patients without risk factors, mortality decreased significantly similar to Boey's [3].

The preoperative shock is associated with a misdiagnosis, late diagnosis, or medical mismanagement; therefore, its reduction depends on medical education.

In terms of diagnosis, experience plays a leading role, and the health organization of many countries means that care services are composed of doctors in training.

3.1.3 Imaging

A simple chest X-ray with visualization of the diaphragmatic domes shows pneumoperitoneum in 65–70% of perforated patients (Popper's sign) (**Figure 9**).

When radiology does not show air in the cavity, it does not invalidate the clinical diagnosis.

If the patient has been perforating for a while and the hemodynamic conditions of the patient make it impossible for him to stand up, a chest X-ray can be performed

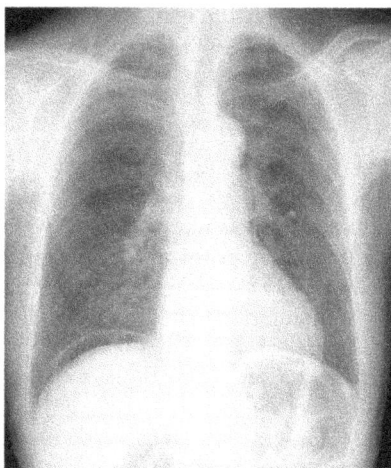

Figure 9.
Frontal chest X-ray. The air bubble below the right hemidiaphragm (on the left of the image) is a pneumoperitoneum.

with the lateral position and the patient in the left lateral decubitus position in order to visualize air between the liver and the chest wall.

When is not found, it may be due to the immediate blockage of perforation by the omentum. It is more frequent in the elderly.

Because pneumoperitoneum is not objectifiable in 30–35% of those perforated, an alternative is pneumogastrophagy, which consists of injecting air into the stomach through the nasogastric tube. In this way, a pneumoperitoneum could become visible and have a more accurate diagnosis, reducing to one-third the time between perforation and surgery and therefore also decreasing mortality to one-third (K. Maull [6]).

3.2 Treatment

The initial management in the perforated PU is the usual performed on every visceral perforation.

Urgent hospitalization in a center with possibilities of laboratory, images, intensive care unit, and eventual surgery. Replacement of fluids with crystalloids and administration of analgesics. Nasogastric tube to reduce the effusion of gastro-duodenal contents to the peritoneum and to evacuate the stomach before a possible emergency surgery. Antibiotics since the diagnosis is made. In case of shock, the placement of a central line, bladder catheter and hospitalization in an intensive care unit, antibiotics, continuous gastric aspiration, and PPIs are added, since the diagnosis of perforation is confirmed.

3.2.1 Surgical treatment

As a fact, every perforation is a surgical treatment emergency with three objectives: closure of the perforation, washing the cavity, and culture of the peritoneal fluid. The classic procedure for closing the perforation is by laparoscopy or laparotomy, making trans-parietal points with resorbable material and omentoplasty if feasible (Graham technique). In the GU, biopsy of the edges is done due to the eventuality of a perforation related to malignancy, but it is also done in the DU to identify HP infection. Laparoscopic treatment is the gold standard [7], and laparotomy is reserved for those patients with general contraindications for laparoscopy as it happens with patients on established shock.

The conversion from laparoscopy to laparotomy rate varies between 0% and 29%, being higher in patients who underwent surgery in shock.

3.2.1.1 Postoperative

The nasogastric tube should remain until intestinal peristalsis is reestablish. The administration of proton pump inhibitors, first intravenous, and then oral should continue until the healing of the ulcer. The presence or absence of H. Pylori is controlled by endoscopy.

At present time with the progress of medical treatment, practically only simple closure of the ulcer is performed [8]. The simple closure is a short and simple operation, and it is available to every surgeon; you can spend more time washing the peritoneal cavity, since peritonitis is the main cause of mortality. It forces a postoperative medical treatment for the possibility of another ulcer of acute lesions, perforation, or bleeding from the sutured ulcer.

3.2.1.2 Complications

Once the acute condition has been treated even with adequate antibiotic coverage, subphrenic abscesses, pelvic abscesses, or between the intestinal loops may be develop.

3.3 Morbidity and mortality

The prognosis of a patient with perforated PU depends on multiple factors:

Age is a non-modifiable factor, and comorbidities can be modified. The doctor is responsible for a quick diagnosis, and the surgeon is responsible of having good training and about choosing an appropriate tactic to each particular case.

Hermon Taylor in 1956 [9] described the nonsurgical treatment of perforated peptic ulcer, in which he considers that aspiration of the nasogastric tube and blocks the perforation with the omentum.

It is not convenient to replace surgery with this method, because more than 25% of patients had to be operated. This method has more complications, longer hospitalization time, and more failure in the elderly. Gastric aspiration is useful in the preoperative or in the period when patients need preoperative stabilization of any previous conditions.

While the patient already diagnosed waits for the surgery and thus by some medical indication (anesthesiologist or other specialist), it is decided to delay it briefly in order to improve some associated disease.

The simplest effective treatment in a perforated peptic ulcer, as soon as possible, is simple closure and lavage of the abdominal cavity.

In summary, mortality in PU perforations for both laparoscopic and laparoscopic surgery remains high and varies between 4.8% and 10.2%.

In order to improve the prognosis in perforated ulcers, we must follow certain statements:

• Culture of the population in order to alert them of symptoms and awareness to hospitals.

• Effective primary care, that is, the first doctor who attends the patient makes an accurate and rapid diagnosis.

- Prompt diagnosis reduces the time until surgical intervention, reducing morbidity and mortality.

- Antibiotic-onset prophylaxis to counteract the progression of infection.

- Emergency surgery and proper operation (limited to simple closure and peritoneal lavage in most cases).

4. Pyloroduodenal obstruction

For many years, pyloroduodenal obstruction (PDO) by peptic ulcer (PU) was one of the classic indications of gastric surgery.

As mentioned in this chapter, the big change occurred by the appearance of H2 blockers and then proton pump inhibitors (PPIs) and eradication of H. Pylori. Before these treatments, the PUs had as a characteristic an extended chronicity.

PDO is always preceded by week or months of dyspepsia. In general, they are progressive and rarely become total because consultations are earlier, except in areas of insufficient medical coverage.

There are two mechanisms of obstruction:

1. By edema and pylorus spams, in active ulcers. They were formerly called "soft pyloric syndromes" because of their good response to medical treatment

2. By the healing of old ulcers, causing fibrosis. They were known as "hard pyloric syndromes" because they did not respond to antiulcer treatment and were surgically indicated.

4.1 Symptomatology

A minority of patients with PU begin their disease with PDO. The first symptoms are usually postprandial fullness for weeks or months. In more advanced stages, there are belching, nausea, and vomiting. The latter usually have traces of food from previous days and generally do not have bile. When provoked, they relieve symptoms immediately.

In cases of gastric retention by an active PU, the classic pain of ulcerative crises is added. In chronic PDO, anorexia leads to malnutrition and persistent vomiting causes dehydration, thirst, and hypokalemic and hypochloremic alkalosis due to the loss of hydrochloric acid and potassium.

4.2 Diagnosis

The symptomatology is so evident, that with the interrogation a diagnosis of gastric retention is made, although the etiology cannot be assured. The physical examination predominates weight loss, dryness of skin, and mucous membranes and oliguria. The abdomen presents with an asymmetrical distension to the left and can reach the pelvis, often with the shape of the distended stomach. Direct radiology of the abdomen shows large gastric dilatation and air liquid interphase characteristic of retention. X-rays contrasted with barium, which used to be routine, are contraindicated before an endoscopy and rarely help to establish the etiological diagnosis. Endoscopy is essential to detect pathology of the esophageal mucosa by reflux, ulcerative lesions of the gastric body, associated with PDO, and discard a carcinoma or other non-ulcerative gastric pathology. In cases of retention due to active ulcers, if the endoscope passes to the duodenum, the need for further dilations decreases.

4.3 Treatment

Medical treatment: The replacement of fluids and electrolytes is a priority due to the abundant loss/lack of intake, meaning the correction of dehydration and the underlying acid-base disorder and in this way permitting the reversion of duodenal edema and transit reestablish. The nasogastric tube should remain as a permanent drain for several days. PPIs are the main medication to maintain a gastric pH > 4.

Endoscopic treatment: The pneumatic dilation of a stenosis due to PU is one of the main advances of the last decade, both for active ulcers and for scars stenosis. In most patients, several dilations are needed. The main risk is perforation, but its incidence is low. Pneumatic dilation is a first line of instrumental therapy, which relieves symptoms and can prevent or defer the need for surgical treatment.

Surgical treatment: Operations, along with the eradication of HP, are the most commonly used treatment. The percentage of patients who are operated is variable and is related to the time of evolution of the PUD. In PDO due to an ulcer in activity it can reach 64%, while in chronic ones with fibrous stenosis it exceeds 98%.

PDO operations are not an emergency and are indicated in clinically compensated patients, which are achieved in the first week before intervention.

The surgery has two objectives. It decreases acid secretion, which is obtained with vagotomy (can be replace by PPI treatment), and improves gastric emptying, with gastrojejunostomy or antral resection.

Postoperative complications are the same as the ones for uncomplicated PU surgery. The most frequent is the delay in evacuation due to gastric hypotonia secondary to prolonged obstruction and usually improves in days or a few weeks.

Acknowledgements

Mario A. Suarez García, Centro de Cirugía de la Obesidad—CCO, Buenos Aires, Argentina, mariosuarezg11@hotmail.com

Claudia A. Refi, Centro de Cirugía de la Obesidad—CCO, Buenos Aires, Argentina, claudiarefi@hotmail.com

Conflict of interest

The authors declare no conflict of interest.

Author details

Carlos A. Casalnuovo[1]*, Pedro A. Brégoli[1], Cesar J. Valdivieso Duarte[2]
and Carlos A. Vera Cedeño[3]

1 Hospital de Clínicas, University of Buenos Aires; Centro de Cirugía de la
Obesidad—CCO, Buenos Aires, Argentina

2 Hospital de Clínicas, University of Buenos Aires, Buenos Aires, Argentina

3 Centro de Cirugía de la Obesidad—CCO, Buenos Aires, Argentina

*Address all correspondence to: cac149@hotmail.com

IntechOpen

References

[1] Rj H, Ls G, Turney EA. Relationship between Helicobacter pylori eradication and reduced duodenal and gastric ulcer recurrence: A review. Gastroenterology. 1996;**110**:1244-1252

[2] Forrest J, Finlayson N, Shearman D. Endoscopy in gastrointestinal bleeding. Lancet. 1974;**2**:394-397

[3] Boey J, Wong J. Perforated duodenal ulcers. World Journal of Surgery. 1987;**11**:319

[4] Casalnuovo C, Montesinos M, Gallo R, Gutierrez V. Factores de riesgo en peritonitis por perforación de úlceras gástricas y duodenales. Revista Argentina de Cirugía. 1989;**57**:134-137

[5] Watkins RM, Dennison AR, Collin J. What has happened to perforated peptic ulcer? The British Journal of Surgery. 1984;**71**:774-776

[6] Maull KI, Reath DB. Pneumogastrography in the diagnosis of perforated peptic ulcer. American Journal of Surgery. 1984;**148**(3):340-345

[7] Lanevicius R, Morkevicius M. Management strategies, early results, benefits and risk factors of laparoscopic repair of perforated peptic ulcer. World Journal of Surgery. 2005;**29**:1299-1310

[8] Rodríguez-Sanjuán JC, Fernández-Santiago R, García RA. Perforated peptic ulcer treated by simple closure and Helicobacter Pylori eradication. World Journal of Surgery. 2005;**29**: 849-852

[9] Hermon TJ, Warren RP. Perforated acute and chronic peptic ulcer conservative treatment. The Lancet. 1956;**267**(6920):397-399

Chapter 4

The Surgical Management of Peptic Ulcer Disease

Gabriela Doyle and Annabel Barber

Abstract

The treatment of peptic ulcer disease has evolved substantially through the decades since the discovery of acid-reducing agents and helicobacter pylori bacteria. With the success of medical treatment, surgical therapy continues to play a less prominent role in the care of this disease. Operative candidates include the naive patient treated with over-the-counter NSAIDs who are often those with undiagnosed Helicobacter pylori, requiring less complicated initial surgery. With more surgeons graduating with less experience operating on PUD with evolving operative techniques, the question arises as to what constitutes the optimal surgical approach, especially in the elective vs. emergent settings. Recent literature discussing GI bleeding associated with COVID-19 also merits discussion of surgical options in this chapter. Future surgical options may include minimally invasive endoscopic surgeries akin to per-oral endoscopic myotomy of the pylorus; however, this has not yet been described in this disease.

Keywords: peptic ulcer disease, Helicobacter pylori, surgical treatment

1. Introduction: The beginnings of peptic ulcer disease surgery and discovery of H. Pylori

Peptic ulcers are not a modern disease. Ulcers have plagued mankind since the age of Hippocrates (born 460 BCE), who had been known to use honey and mastic oil for symptomatic relief. Record of surgery for a gastric ulcer was found written in stone in the temple of Aesculapius at Epidaurus as described by Goldstein in 1943: "A man with an ulcer in his stomach…Asklepios opened his stomach, cut out the ulcer, sewed him up again, and loosed his bonds. He went away whole, but the chamber was covered with his blood" [1], (Goldstein HI. Ulcer and cancer of the stomach in the middle ages. J Internal Coll Surgeons. 1943;**6**:482–489.) Millenia would pass by before Polish surgeon, Dr. Ludwik Rydygier, would begin the era of modern peptic ulcer surgery. In 1881, Rydygier performed the first successful antral resection for a gastric ulcer penetrating to the pancreas. Rydygier would go on to advocate for resection in the treatment of gastric ulcers in cases characterized by perforation or bleeding, and for antral cancer. The gastroenterostomy too was pioneered by Rydygier, performed for the first time by the Polish surgeon on a patient with a duodenal ulcer [2].

Exactly 100 years after Rydygier's groundbreaking surgery, pathologist Dr. Robin Warren met Dr. Barry Marshall at the Royal Perth Hospital, Australia during internal medicine fellowship training. Sharing an interest in the physiology of gastritis, they spent 2 years studying the stomach and discovered the spiral bacteria *H. pylori*. Marshall and Warren developed the hypothesis that this bacterium played a role of the development of peptic ulcers. The pair went so far as to drink solution containing H. Pylori, predicting eventual ulcer development, and discovering in the following weeks that H. pylori had colonized the stomach and caused gastritis [3]. While initially met with some skepticism, the link between H. pylori and peptic ulcer disease served a pioneering discovery that changed the treatment for PUD and earned Marshall and Warren the Nobel Prize in Medicine in 2005 [4].

In the wake of Marshall and Warren's achievement, new therapies evolved against peptic ulcer disease. Proposed treatments have been published since the 1990s and updated to reflect the advancements in diagnostics, resistance to antibiotics, and geographic prevalence patterns. General regimens include acid-reducing agents and various antimicrobials [1]. Medical therapy has proven to be largely successful in combating H. Pylori, with eradication rates of 70–95% across several trials [5, 6]. The patterns of peptic ulcer disease have therefore shifted from a once-common surgical problem to an entity treated effectively through oral medications.

2. The relevance of invasive intervention for PUD in 2020s

Several studies have shown that hospitalizations for peptic ulcer disease have declined since the 1980s [7–10]. However, despite improvement due much in part to the advancement of medical therapy, PUD persists in the population with a lifetime prevalence in of 5–10% and incidence of 0.1–0.3% yearly. Roughly 10–20% of these patients experience complications, including hemorrhage and less commonly, perforation [11]. The sequelae of PUD complications are often life-threatening and it is in these cases that surgical evaluation must be sought.

The current role for surgery in peptic ulcer disease is largely in the emergent setting, with bleeding, perforation, and obstruction as the major indications for intervention.

3. Operative approach: perforated peptic ulcers

In patients with perforated peptic ulcer disease with significant pneumoperitoneum, extraluminal contrast extravasation on diagnostic study, or signs of peritonitis, operative treatment is recommended [11]. It is further suggested that the operation is performed promptly (within 24 hours) to decrease morbidity and mortality [12, 13]. Endoscopy currently has no role in the treatment of acutely perforated peptic ulcers. The laparoscopic and open approaches have both been described in the management of perforated peptic ulcers. Selection of surgical approach is based at least partially on surgeon experience and available equipment. In unstable patients, open surgery is favored. Several studies have pointed to comparable outcomes between open and laparoscopic surgery including overall postoperative complication rate, mortality, and reoperation rate. Laparoscopic surgery may have advantages in reducing hospital stay, lowering rate of surgical site infection, and less postoperative pain when compared to open surgery [14–16]. Robotic-assisted laparoscopic surgery has not been widely used for perforated or bleeding peptic ulcers and is not currently recommended in an emergent setting.

Several factors will tailor the ultimate surgical intervention to be performed. These include ulcer location, ulcer size, history of prior surgeries, prior ulcer treatment and patient stability. With gastric ulcers, excision of the ulcer with reconstruction of the resultant defect is the operative goal. For gastric ulcers located in the greater curvature, antrum, or body of the stomach, a wedge excision of the ulcer usually can be performed easily with linear staplers. Wedge resection results in both closure of the perforation and obtaining a tissue sample for biopsy—a critical consideration give the reported 4–14% rate of malignancy in perforated gastric ulcers [17]. Ulcers along the lesser curvature present a challenge given the proximity to the GE junction and the left gastric arterial flow. In distal lesser curvature ulcer cases, a distal gastrectomy may be considered. The proximal ulcer close to the gastroesophageal junction may require a subtotal gastrectomy with a subsequent Roux-en-Y esophagogastrojejunostomy.

It is important to note that perforations of the pyloric channel and the duodenum are functionally grouped together. Treatment of a small perforated duodenal ulcers (<2 cm) classically involves pedicled omentum placed into the defect as a repair. Primary repair, with or without an omental patch has also been described. Historically, an omental patch has been advocated to buttress a primary repair; however, recent studies point to no meaningful difference in leakage rate or mortality with addition of this step [18]. The operative approach to larger duodenal ulcers requires thorough calculation and a large range of interventions are available based on each patient's individual scenario. An omental patch repair in duodenal ulcer perforations that are greater than 2 cm in size have an increased rate of postoperative leaks (up to 12%) [17]. Partial gastrectomy with subsequent reconstruction via a gastroduodenostomy (Billroth I) or gastrojejunostomy (Billroth II) may be performed to address the ulcer and restore gastrointestinal continuity. Additionally, the jejunum can be used in a pedicled graft or serosal patch approach. The involvement of the duodenum containing the ampulla of Vater is a particularly arduous challenge. When in doubt, the integrity of the ampulla should be investigated with intraoperative cholangiography. Damage-control procedures such as the Roux-en-Y duodenojejunostomy or pyloric exclusion may be warranted in patients with tenuous stability. The duodenostomy tube should be considered as last-resort procedure when the patient's hemodynamic status on the operating table will not allow for a more complex operation. An emergent Whipple comes with a high rate of morbidity and mortality and should generally not be attempted.

4. Operative approach: bleeding peptic ulcers

The evolution of endoscopic skills and technology in the last several decades has brought this technique to the forefront of bleeding ulcers and often obviates the need for surgical intervention. Early endoscopy (within 24 hours) is first-line therapy with the employment of therapeutic endoscopic interventions as needed, along with the initiation of parenteral proton pump inhibitors [11]. Roughly 10–20% of patients will have recurrent bleeding despite endoscopic therapy, at which time repeat endoscopy should be considered [19]. Patients who remain hemodynamically stable thereafter without high-risk ulcer features may then be safely discharged with continued oral PPI management. Surgery becomes warranted in cases of bleeding peptic ulcers when endoscopy fails or when the patient is deemed high-risk of a rebleeding event. Large ulcers (>2 cm) and hypotension at rebleeding are reported independent factors of predicting failure in further endoscopic treatment. Other features reported to prompt surgical consultation for further management include pulsatile bleeding, visible blood vessels in posterior duodenal ulcers, and transfusion requirement greater than 6 units of blood in the first 24 hours [20].

The surgical procedures currently used in bleeding gastroduodenal ulcers are on a spectrum of minimal to definitive interventions. The principal objective in life-saving surgery is hemorrhage control, which may be achieved through simple intraluminal oversewing or ligature, plication, or excision of the ulcer and repair of the defect [20]. The initial procedure may also include control of the arteries of the stomach or duodenum through direct ligation.

5. The role of acid-reducing procedures

The management of emergent PUD has largely left out procedures that were designed to address the underlying problem--a once common consideration in all patients with PUD up until the 20th century. Acid-reducing procedures histori-cally included division of the vagus nerve at various points in order to decrease the acetylcholine-mediated secretion of acid from parietal cells [21].

The truncal vagotomy is the division of the anterior and posterior trunks of the vagus nerves roughly 4 cm proximal to the gastro-esophageal junction. Stimulation of parietal cells is interrupted through this procedure; however, the lack of sympa-thetic input to the stomach results in a lack of relaxation, thereby decreasing the propulsion of solids from the stomach into the small intestine. Therefore, a concom-itant drainage procedure, consisting of a pyloroplasty or antral resection would be performed. A selective vagotomy is similar but involves division of the vagus nerves at the more distal anterior and posterior branches after the level of the celiac and hepatobiliary branching. The highly selective vagotomy (HSV) was tailored to avoid the need for a drainage procedure. The HSV involves division of the nerve fibers supplying the parietal cells of the fundus and body of stomach, sparing the "crows's foot" fibers innervating the antrum and pylorus. Given the rise of medical manage-ment, the role of the vagotomy with or without drainage procedures in peptic ulcer disease is limited to very few cases [22].

The main indication for consideration of an acid-reducing procedure are patients whose disease is refractory to medical management or those who cannot reliably participate or tolerate proton-pump inhibitors. Specifically, it is cases of duodenal ulcers (Type II and III) in which a vagotomy may be considered--gastric ulcers (TYpe I, IV) are not related to acid hypersecretion and therefore resection alone is indicated. In emergent situations, including bleeding duodenal ulcers and perforated duodenal ulcers, the use of a vagotomy is debated and is often surgeon-dependent. In general, the presence of peritonitis, shock, abdominal abscess, delay in treatment over 24 hours, or severe concurrent medical illness are contraindica-tions to lengthening the surgery by adding a vagotomy to the rest of the surgical management plan [22, 23].

6. Future surgical considerations

In the era of rapidly advancing surgical instruments and techniques, innovations in peptic ulcer disease surgery are rising in efforts to improve patient outcomes. The robotic platform is emerging as a feasible alternative to surgical treatment in the elective settings for many diseases. There have a been case reports of gastric resec-tions performed safely with the assistance of the surgical robot, and whether the robot has a wider role for peptic ulcer disease merits exploration [24, 25]. Most prior reports of robotic assisted laparoscopic surgery for the stomach are those done for malignancy.

The pedicled omental plug for a large duodenal ulcer is a described twist on the classic omental patch closure. In this procedure, a nasogastric tube is inserted through the oropharynx and down through the perforation. A tongue of omentum is then secured to the tube via sutures and withdrawn into the stomach, where it is sutured to the ulcer edges. This omental plug shows promise, as was associated with a lower recurrent leak and duodenal stenosis rate in a randomized trial comparison against the standard omental patch [26]. Falciform flaps may be a feasible option in patients who do not have a viable omentum [27].

7. PUD and the advent of COVID-19

With the introduction of SARS-CoV-2 to the world's collective biome we have observed unprecedented patterns of illness, with both the aversion of presenting to an affected hospital and the virus itself affecting disease across multiple organ systems. We here present a look at the relationship, if any, between COVID-19 and peptic ulcer disease.

It is well-known that COVID-19 presents with respiratory symptoms; however, several other manifestations are being seen. In one study comprised of over 20,000 patients, up to 29% had enteric symptoms including abdominal pain, nausea, vomiting, and diarrhea [28]. The pathophysiology of gastrointestinal tract mani-festations of COVID-19 is thought to stem from several biochemical mechanisms including infection of the GI tract/liver leading to cellular inflammation and damage, dysbiosis enhancing the inflammatory response and cytokine storm, and affliction of the neuroenteric system [29].

GI bleeding is a reported, though less common manifestation associated with COVID-19. A rather high prevalence of PUD complicated by bleeding was noticed in one cohort of patients with moderate-to-severe ARDs caused by COVID-19 [29]. In another study performed on COVID-positive hospitalized patients undergoing endoscopy (n = 106), one-fourth of the studied population had peptic ulcers while an additional 16% had erosive/ulcerative gastro-duodenopathy [30]. The mainstay of treat-ment in peptic ulcer disease is proton-pump inhibitors; however, at least one study has demonstrated that PPI treatment is associated with worse outcomes in those infected by SARS-CoV-2 and development of COVID-19 when compared to individuals who are not taking a PPI [28]. The mechanism responsible for this finding remains unclear.

Another factor to consider in patients afflicted with peptic ulcer disease is the pattern of behavior in seeking medical evaluation during a pandemic. As the admissions for COVID-19 related respiratory illnesses increased dramatically, several hospitals reported decreased admissions and emergency medicine visits for non-COVID related diseases [31–33]. Theories concerning this trends in admissions during the pandemic include failure to present to a hospital secondary to fear of contracting COVID-19, which may have made some cases of illness more profound up to the point of death in the community [33]. The first United States Coronavirus epicenter in New York performed a multicenter study looking specifically at emer-gent general surgery admissions. Comparison to prior years indicated that there was an overall decrease in admissions with an overall increase in mortality. Peptic ulcer disease was one of the seven diagnoses that was observed [34]. A delay of 12 hours was found in 10 cases of complicated peptic ulcer disease in one institution during a two-month period [35]. The question arises if the increase in mortality is at least in part attributable to delayed presentation.

The full clinical spectrum of COVID-19 has not yet fully been elucidated. There is surprisingly limited data on the relationship between COVID-19 and peptic ulcer disease. The pathogenesis of ulcers in the setting of SARS-CoV-2 affliction may be related to direct gastric epithelial damage, stress resulting from the acute disease, or active mucosal inflammation sustained by cytokine storming [36]. Development of treatment guidelines in COVID-19 positive patients who sustain gastrointestinal manifestations of disease warrants further investigation.

8. Final reflections

Peptic ulcer disease remains a healthcare issue across the world and requires an interdisciplinary approach. In linking H. Pylori and NSAID use to peptic ulcers, pioneering efforts in controlling PUD have largely been seen in the primary care setting. However, complications from PUD persist in the population, and surgical intervention will continue to play a role in the very worst of the disease burden. It is therefore the responsibility of the surgical community to advance care through innovation of technique to provide optimal outcomes. This is especially true in the era of a pandemic where healthcare dynamics are adversely affected.

Author details

Gabriela Doyle and Annabel Barber*
The Kirk Kerkorian School of Medicine, Las Vegas, USA

*Address all correspondence to: annabelbarber@gmail.com

IntechOpen

References

[1] Matsumoto H, Shiotani A, Graham DY. Current and future treatment of helicobacter pylori infections. Advances in Experimental Medicine and Biology. 2019;**1149**:211-225. DOI: 10.1007/5584_2019_367

[2] Pach R, Orzel-Nowak A, Scully T. Ludwik Rydygier--contributor to modern surgery. Gastric Cancer. 2008;**11**(4):187-191. DOI: 10.1007/s10120-008-0482-7

[3] Marshall BJ, Armstrong JA, McGechie DB, Clancy RJ. Attempt to fulfil Koch's postulates for pyloric Campylobacter. The Medical Journal of Australia. 1985;**142**(8):436-439. DOI: 10.5694/j.1326-5377.1985.tb113443.x

[4] The Nobel Prize in Physiology or Medicine 2005. NobelPrize.org. https://www.nobelprize.org/prizes/medicine/2005/7693-the-nobel-prize-in-physiology-or-medicine-2005-2005-6/ [Accessed: 08 September 2021]

[5] Fennerty MB, Lieberman DA, Vakil N, Magaret N, Faigel DO, Helfand M. Effectiveness of helicobacter pylori therapies in a clinical practice setting. Archives of Internal Medicine. 1999;**159**(14):1562-1566. DOI: 10.1001/archinte.159.14.1562

[6] Rokkas T, Gisbert JP, Malfertheiner P, et al. Comparative effectiveness of multiple different first-line treatment regimens for helicobacter pylori infection: A network meta-analysis. Gastroenterology. 2021;**161**(2):495-507. e4. DOI: 10.1053/j.gastro.2021.04.012

[7] Lewis JD, Bilker WB, Brensinger C, Farrar JT, Strom BL. Hospitalization and mortality rates from peptic ulcer disease and GI bleeding in the 1990s: Relationship to sales of nonsteroidal anti-inflammatory drugs and acid suppression medications. The American Journal of Gastroenterology.

2002;**97**(10):2540-2549. DOI: 10.1111/j.1572-0241.2002.06037.x

[8] Post PN, Kuipers EJ, Meijer GA. Declining incidence of peptic ulcer but not of its complications: A nation-wide study in The Netherlands. Alimentary Pharmacology & Therapeutics. 2006;**23**(11):1587-1593. DOI: 10.1111/j.1365-2036.2006.02918.x

[9] Feinstein LB, Holman RC, Christensen KLY, Steiner CA, Swerdlow DL. Trends in hospitalizations for peptic ulcer disease, United States, 1998-2005. Emerging Infectious Diseases Journal - CDC. 2010;**16**(9): 1410-1418. DOI: 10.3201/eid1609.091126

[10] El-Serag HB, Sonnenberg A. Opposing time trends of peptic ulcer and reflux disease. Gut. 1998;**43**(3):327-333. DOI: 10.1136/gut.43.3.327

[11] Tarasconi A, Coccolini F, Biffl WL, et al. Perforated and bleeding peptic ulcer: WSES guidelines. World Journal of Emergency Surgery : WJES. 2020;**15**:3. DOI: 10.1186/s13017-019-0283-9

[12] Buck DL, Vester-Andersen M, Møller MH. Danish clinical register of emergency surgery. Surgical delay is a critical determinant of survival in perforated peptic ulcer. The British Journal of Surgery. 2013;**100**(8):1045-1049. DOI: 10.1002/bjs.9175

[13] Møller MH, Adamsen S, Thomsen RW, Møller AM. Preoperative prognostic factors for mortality in peptic ulcer perforation: A systematic review. Scandinavian Journal of Gastroenterology. 2010;**45**(7-8):785-805. DOI: 10.3109/00365521003783320

[14] Siow SL, Mahendran HA, Wong CM, Hardin M, Luk TL. Laparoscopic versus open repair of perforated peptic ulcer: Improving

outcomes utilizing a standardized technique. Asian Journal of Surgery. 2018;**41**(2):136-142. DOI: 10.1016/j.asjsur.2016.11.004

[15] Tan S, Wu G, Zhuang Q, et al. Laparoscopic versus open repair for perforated peptic ulcer: A meta analysis of randomized controlled trials. International Journal of Surgery. 2016;**33**(Pt A):124-132. DOI: 10.1016/j.ijsu.2016.07.077

[16] Zhou C, Wang W, Wang J, et al. An updated meta-analysis of laparoscopic versus open repair for perforated peptic ulcer. Scientific Reports. 2015;**5**(1): 13976. DOI: 10.1038/srep13976

[17] Lee CW, Sarosi GA. Emergency ulcer surgery. The Surgical Clinics of North America. 2011;**91**(5):1001-1013. DOI: 10.1016/j.suc.2011.06.008

[18] Lo H-C, Wu S-C, Huang H-C, Yeh C-C, Huang J-C, Hsieh C-H. Laparoscopic simple closure alone is adequate for low risk patients with perforated peptic ulcer. World Journal of Surgery. 2011;**35**(8):1873-1878. DOI: 10.1007/s00268-011-1106-7

[19] Banerjee S, Cash BD, Dominitz JA, et al. The role of endoscopy in the management of patients with peptic ulcer disease. Gastrointestinal Endoscopy. 2010;**71**(4):663-668. DOI: 10.1016/j.gie.2009.11.026

[20] Abe N, Takeuchi H, Yanagida O, Sugiyama M, Atomi Y. Surgical indications and procedures for bleeding peptic ulcer. Digestive Endoscopy. 2010;**22**(s1):S35-S37. DOI: 10.1111/j.1443-1661.2010.00966.x

[21] Lagoo J, Pappas TN, Perez A. A relic or still relevant: The narrowing role for vagotomy in the treatment of peptic ulcer disease. American Journal of Surgery. 2014;**207**(1):120-126. DOI: 10.1016/j.amjsurg.2013.02.012

[22] Seeras K, Qasawa RN, Prakash S. Truncal vagotomy. In: StatPearls. StatPearls Publishing; 2021. Available from: http://www.ncbi.nlm.nih.gov/books/NBK526104/ [Accessed: 26 September 2021]

[23] Feliciano DV. Do perforated duodenal ulcers need an acid-decreasing surgical procedure now that omeprazole is available? The Surgical Clinics of North America. 1992;**72**(2):369-380. DOI: 10.1016/s0039-6109(16)45684-7

[24] Omental Patch Repair For Perforated Duodenal Ulcer: Robotic Approach In A Patient With Delayed Presentation - SAGES Abstract Archives. SAGES. Available from: https://www.sages.org/meetings/annual-meeting/abstracts-archive/omental-patch-repair-for-perforated-duodenal-ulcerrobotic-approach-in-a-patient-with-delayed-presentation/ [Accessed: 17 September 2021]

[25] Robotic Distal Gastrectomy for refractory peptic ulcer disease - SAGES Abstract Archives. SAGES. Available from: https://www.sages.org/meetings/annual-meeting/abstracts-archive/robotic-distal-gastrectomy-for-refractory-peptic-ulcer-disease/ [Accessed: 17 September 2021]

[26] Jani K, Saxena AK, Vaghasia R. Omental plugging for large-sized duodenal peptic perforations: A prospective randomized study of 100 patients. Southern Medical Journal. 2006;**99**(5):467-471. DOI: 10.1097/01.smj.0000203814.87306.cd

[27] Ahmadinejad M, Maghsoudi L. Novel approach for peptic ulcer perforation surgery. Clinical Case Reports. 2020;**8**:1937-1939. DOI: 10.1002/ccr3.3030

[28] Hunt RH, East JE, Lanas A, et al. COVID-19 and Gastrointestinal Disease: Implications for the Gastroenterologist. Digestive Diseases. Published online

October. 2020;**9**:1-21. DOI: 10.1159/000512152

[29] Marasco G, Lenti MV, Cremon C, et al. Implications of SARS-CoV-2 infection for neurogastroenterology. Neurogastroenterology and Motility. 2021;**33**(3):141-144. DOI: 10.1111/nmo.14104

[30] Vanella G, Capurso G, Burti C, et al. Gastrointestinal mucosal damage in patients with COVID-19 undergoing endoscopy: an international multicentre study. BMJ Open Gastroenterology. 2021;**8**(1):e000578. DOI: 10.1136/bmjgast-2020-000578

[31] Rennert-May E, Leal J, Thanh NX, et al. The impact of COVID-19 on hospital admissions and emergency department visits: A population-based study. PLoS One. 2021;**16**(6):e0252441. DOI: 10.1371/journal.pone.0252441

[32] Heist T, Schwartz K. Trends in Overall and Non-COVID-19 Hospital Admissions. KFF. 2021. Available from: https://www.kff.org/health-costs/issue-brief/trends-in-overall-and-non-covid-19-hospital-admissions/ [Accessed: 17 September 2021]

[33] Shoaib A, Van Spall HGC, Wu J, et al. Substantial decline in hospital admissions for heart failure accompanied by increased community mortality during COVID-19 pandemic. European Heart Journal - Quality of Care & Clinical Outcomes. 2021;**7**(4):378-387. DOI: 10.1093/ehjqcco/qcab040

[34] Dong CT, Liveris A, Lewis ER, et al. Do surgical emergencies stay at home? Observations from the first United States coronavirus epicenter. Journal of Trauma and Acute Care Surgery. 2021;**91**(1):241-246. DOI: 10.1097/TA.0000000000003202

[35] Bagus BI. Predictor factor for inpatients mortality of peptic ulcer emergency surgery during COVID-19 pandemic. International Journal of Surgery Science. 2021;**5**(2):211-213. DOI: 10.33545/surgery.2021.v5.i2d.693

[36] Melazzini F, Lenti MV, Mauro A, De Grazia F, Di Sabatino A. Peptic ulcer disease as a common cause of bleeding in patients with coronavirus disease. The American Journal of Gastroenterology. Published online May 22, 2020. 2019;**115**:1139-1140. DOI: 10.14309/ajg.0000000000000710

Vonoprazan Versus Conventional Proton Pump Inhibitor in the Therapeutic Armamentarium of Peptic Ulcer Disease and Gastroesophageal Reflux Disease

Radu Seicean

Abstract

Vonoprazan is a novel potassium-competitive acid blocker that has been introduced as an effective treatment option in peptic ulcer and gastroesophageal reflux diseases. Its adverse events panel is encouraging compared to standard proton pump inhibitors, although higher hypergastrinemia and foveolar-type gastric adenocarcinoma occurrence have been described. The efficiency is proved in gastric and duodenal ulcer, gastroesophageal reflux and gastric post- endoscopic submucosal dissection ulcers, with higher ulcer shrinkage rate and no incremental risk for bleeding. The new therapies containing Vonoprazan instead of convention proton pump inhibitors against Helicobacter pylori are safe and well-tolerated, being associated with a better eradication rate. However, the therapy should be adjusted to the body size.

Keywords: Vonoprazan, Helicobacter pylori, peptic ulcer, proton pump inhibitors, gastroesophageal reflux

1. Introduction

Vonoprazan is part of the potassium competitive acid blockers (P-CABs) family that has been reported as being effective against a range of stomach acid related conditions due to its acid suppressant activity. It activates on the final step of the acid secretion pathway, more specifically on the gastric $H+/K + -ATPase$ proton pump. Due to its effects as an acid suppressor, vonoprazan is reported as being useful in preventing acid-related injuries due to excessive acid exposure. Pathologies, where such effects may prove useful, include gastroesophageal reflux disease (GERD), peptic ulcer disease (PUD) as well as infections with *Helicobacter Pylori* [1].

2. Methodology

We performed an extensive search of PubMed using the following terms: vonoprazan, ulcer peptic disease, gastroesophageal reflux disease, Helicobacter pylori, NSAIDs, submucosal dissection limited to randomized controlled trials, multicenter studies, observational studies, and controlled or uncontrolled clinical trials. We applied filters for the English language and for the adult population.

3. Drug comparison

Vonoprazan, unavailable in Europe and USA, is classed as P-CABs that selectively bind to the E2-P conformation of H+/K + -ATPase inhibit K + -stimulated acid secretion by competing with K+ in binding to E2-P. Together with proton pump inhibitors (PPI) are the drugs used to treat acid-related diseases because of their inhibiting action on H+/K + -ATPase. There are several differences in behavior and characteristics between these two drug categories. Vonoprazan has an ionic and reversible binding method which is different from the covalent and irreversible binding of proton pump inhibitors (PPI). It can link with H+/K + -ATPase in both active and rest phases, meanwhile, the PPIs act only on the active phase. It is also acid-stable, unlike PPIs, and it has a greater half-life (9 hours) as opposed to PPIs (0.5–2.1 hours). Its potency of inhibition is 350 times higher than lansoprazole.

Vonoprazan is absorbed rapidly and reaches maximum plasma concentration at 1.5–2.0 h after oral administration. Food has minimal effect on its intestinal absorption. The mean apparent terminal half-life of the drug is approximately 7.7 h in healthy adults. Vonoprazan is metabolized to inactive metabolites mainly by cytochrome P4502. The plasma protein binding of vonoprazan is 80% in healthy subjects. It distributes extensively into tissues with a mean apparent volume of distribution of 1050 L. This aids in vonoprazan's greater ease of use because it only requires only one administration to be effective and it is also flexible in its administration time, allowing for after meal administration in contrast to PPIs which require not only repeated administration but also strict before meal administration. It has also been observed that Vonoprazan administration leads to a significantly higher pH value (9.06) than PPIs (3.8–5.0). There is no correlation observed between median intragastric pH and CYP2C19 genotypes [1].

4. Role of vonoprazan in gastric/duodenal ulcer

Because vonoprazan elicited a more extensive gastric acid suppression than the proton pump inhibitor, lansoprazole, it also gave rise to two to three times greater serum gastrin concentrations as compared with lansoprazole. During repeated dosing of 20 mg once daily, the 24-h intragastric pH >4 holding time ratios were 63 and 83% on days 1 and 7, respectively [2]. Vonoprazan is recommended by Japanese guidelines for healing gastric /duodenal ulcer as an alternative to PPI, both being superior to anti H2 treatment [3].

5. Efficiency in use for post-endoscopic submucosal dissection (ESD) ulcers

5.1 Vonoprazan vs. esomeprazole

The first study that is to be discussed is a controlled test between a mix of Vonoprazan versus Esomeprazole in treating ESD-induced ulcers. Esomeprazole is a PPI, that is reported to have shown greater inhibitory action than other PPIs. This study used patients who had undergone ESD for gastric neoplasm and excluded and who were either allergic to the medicine or had a severe heart or liver disfunction. The *H. pylori* patients received eradication therapy after the trial.

Out of a total of 84 patients, 40 were randomly assigned to the 20 mg Esomeprazole group and 44 to the 20 mg Vonoprazan group. Two patients could not complete the study, so the analysis was based on the remaining 43 patients in the Vonoprazan group and the 39 in the Esomeprazole group.

In the end, this study yielded no significant results that confirmed a difference between the two treatment options. At 4 weeks, the Vonoprazan group had an ulcer scar rate of 20.9% and a size reduction rate of 94.6%. Meanwhile, the Esomeprazole group had an ulcer scar rate of 15.4% and a size reduction rate of 93.8%. At the 8-week point, the ulcer scar rate for the Vonoprazan group was 90.7% and 92.3% for the Esomeprazole group. The ulcer reduction rates were 99.7% for the Vonoprazan group and 99.3% for the Esomeprazole group.

Delayed bleeding occurred in one patient from the Vonoprazan group and 4 of the Esomeprazole group (2.33% and 10.2%, respectively). No perforations occurred in either group and while there was one case of Mallory-Weiss syndrome in the Esomeprazole group and one case of acute myocardial infarction in the Vonoprazan group, the incidence of these conditions poses no statistical difference between the two drugs. As well as that, no adverse effects regarding the drugs used in the study were observed [4].

5.2 *Vonoprazan* vs. *lansoprazole*

The study drew patients from a population of Japanese natives treated with gastric neoplasm by use of ESD. They were then randomly distributed across two groups that were to be treated either with vonoprazan 20 mg (61 patients-V groups) or lansoprazole 30 mg (66 patients- L group).

The healing ratio at 4 and 8 weeks did not differ significantly between the V and L groups was statistically insignificant.

Delayed bleeding was observed in both groups of patients with no statistical difference between them. Perforation was observed in one patient from the V group and two patients from the L group [5].

Other randomized controlled trial on 216 patients evaluated the healing effects of vonoprazan and lansoprazole on ESD-induced ulcers. Again, there were no significant differences in the reduction rate of ulcers between the vonoprazan and lansoprazole groups at 4 weeks, 94.0 vs. 93.4% or 8 weeks, 99.8 vs. 99.9% [6].

5.3 *Vonoprazan* vs. *Rabeprazole*

From 190 patients who underwent ESD, there were 167 enrolled in the study, being split into a Rabeprazole group (n = 90), which received 20 mg rabeprazole orally once per day, and a V group (n = 77) which received 20 mg vonoprazan orally once per day.

The efficiency evaluation was done based on the healing ratio between vonoprazan and rabeprazole groups as well as the scarring ratio between the two groups.

The scarring rates of all lesions were not significantly different between the vonoprazan and rabeprazole groups (31.7 vs. 18.9%; p = 0.07). There were exceptions for lesions with a diameter ≤ 35 mm. For this category scarring rate in the vonoprazan group was superior to that in the rabeprazole group (42.2 vs. 19.2%; p < 0.05). This was also the case for ulcers with a surface lesser than 3–100 mm2, for which scarring rate in the vonoprazan group also was superior to that in the rabeprazole group (48.7 vs. 20.0%; p < 0.05).

Overall, the reduction rate for all lesions was superior in the V group (93.0 vs. 90.4%; p < 0.05), being distributed similarly to the scarring rates, meaning that lesions under 35 mm in diameter and 3–100 mm^2 are shown to have superior healing times in the V group than in the R group. However, for those lesions greater than these, there have been no statistical differences in the reduction rates between groups.

It was also found that Vonoprazan is superior to Rabeprazole for compete for ulcer scarring (OR 2.21; 95% CI 1.03–4.71; p < 0.05), therefore reducing the risk of incomplete scarring for large lesions.

Further complications, such as delayed bleeding were found in both groups, but their distribution was statistically insignificant [7].

A meta-analysis study including (5 studies, 2 abstracts) patient's healing rates at 4 and 8 weeks post-ESD was conducted in the early days of Vonoprazan's introduction in Japan had shown that a 20 mg Vonoprazan dose had similar treatment efficiency to standard PPI based treatment schemes [8].

Later on, another meta-analysis study was performed, also utilizing studies based on Japanese subjects, which showed significant results when comparing Vonoprazan with other PPI based treatments. In the end, six studies were selected. Initial results at a period between 4 and 8 weeks post ESD showed that the OR for complete healing in patients treated with Vonoprazan stood at 2.27 when compared with patients treated with PPIs. The statistical heterogeneity was insignificant, with an I2 of 0%. Subgroup analysis based on the time of repeated upper endoscopy yielded a significantly higher rate of completely healed ulcers in both the 4-week and the 8-week subgroup, with pooled ORs of 2.21 and 2.40, respectively. This meta-analysis has also shown that while the OR (0.79) of adverse effects is numerically lower for vonoprazan than PPI, statistical analysis has not been shown to be statistically relevant [9].

Another meta-analysis on 1328 patients showed a potential superiority on reducing the risk of post-ESD bleeding compared with PPIs, with a pooled OR of 0.69, although there was no statistically significant difference, with a higher scar formation rate OR = 1.58 [10]. Therefore, it is conclusive to state that Vonoprazan is a superior treatment method in case of post-ESD ulcers, especially in the first 2 weeks of treatment [11] and its side effects are no more severe than other PPI based treatments [12].

The bleeding rate in post ESD 1715 patients was lower for vonoprazan than PPI with an overall bleeding: 11.9% vs. 17.2%, p = 0.008; bleeding between days 2 and 30: 7.8% vs. 11.8%, p = 0.015 and readmission rate for bleeding 2.4% vs. 4.1%, p = 0.081 in a retrospective study [13]. A prospective multicentric Japanese study showed that the rate of delayed bleeding in the Vonoprazan and PPI groups was 3.9 and 4.4%, respectively with non-inferiority for the scar-stage ulcer at 6 weeks in the Vonoprazan group and 8 weeks in the PPI group was 68.3 and 74.6%, respectively (p = 0.19) [14].

6. Vonoprazan in the treatment of *H. pylori*

The triple therapy using PPI/amoxicillin/metronidazole or PPI/amoxicillin/clarithromycine or PPI based quadruple (bismuth salt/tetracycline/nitro-imidazol) is associated with an 80–92% eradication rate [3]. The association of Vonoprazan with different antibiotics for HP eradication showed a high rate of eradication (97%) and in the patients who had prior treatments for HP, the non- vonoprazan therapy was associated with a lower eradication rate (91%) [15]. A multicentric randomized study proved that the 7-day vonoprazan and low-dose amoxicillin dual therapy provided acceptable *H. pylori* eradication rates and a similar effect to vonoprazan-based triple therapy in regions with high clarithromycin resistance (eradication rate of 84.5% and 89.2%) [16]. A recent meta-analysis showed that the best results for HP eradication were obtained with vonoprazan triple therapy, over 90%, and the standard triple therapy had the lowest results [17]. The recommendation of the 2020 guideline sustains the use of vonoprazan as first line therapy, using antibiotics such as amoxicillin, clarithromycin, or metronidazole [3]. When PPI is used as first-line therapy, the indication is to use quadruple therapy or sequential therapy [18]. For the second-line therapy, the association of PPI or Vonoprazan with amoxyciline and metrondazol is recommended [3]. Also, the incidence of adverse events in vonoprazan-based triple therapy was lower than that in PPI-based triple therapy (pooled incidence, 32.7% vs. 40.5% [19].

Successful H. pylori eradication with vonoprazan- amoxicillin dual therapy was associated with the small body size of patients (eradication rate: 90.8% in patients with body surface area < 1.723 vs. 79.6% in those with body surface area ≥ 1.723; p = 0.045). This showed that vonoprazan therapy should be adjusted to body size [20].

The impact of the therapy of eradication based on Vonoprazan was studied in 43 patients in association with Amoxicillin or Amoxicylin/ Claritromicine. One year assessment of gut microbiota was modified qualitatively and quantitatively and correlations with the bodyweight were found [21].

7. Drug-induced ulcers

Vonoprazan is not recommended yet for treating ulcers that occurred after NSAIDS when the interruption of NSAIDs and association with PPI is considered, but they are recommended for their prevention [3].

7.1 Ulcer recurrence prevention during long term NSAID therapy

Those patients that receive NSAID treatment for chronic illnesses to manage inflammatory symptoms have been found to have a risk of ulcers as high as 62%. The current solution for patients that need this treatment is to prescribe acid blockers alongside the treatment.

One randomized controlled study compared Lansoprazol 15 mg with Vonoprazan 10 mg and 20 mg in patients under NSAIDs treatment but with no history of ulcer.

There were non-inferiority effects of Vonoprazan 10 mg and 20 mg when compared to the lansoprazole 15 mg group. Recurrent peptic ulcers within 24 weeks on endoscopy assessment were lower for the vonoprazan 10 mg (3.3%) and 20 mg (3.4%) groups compared with the lansoprazole 15 mg group (5.5%). The non-inferiority effect of vonoprazan 10 mg and 20 mg to lansoprazole was verified because the percentage difference between treatment groups was <8.3% (percentage difference − 2.2%, p < 0.001; −2.1%, p < 0.001, respectively). Tolerability was not apparent to be related to the dosage in Vonoprazan patients [22]. In conclusion, in NSAIDs patients, the use of VPZ is recommended for the prevention of ulcer recurrence.

7.2 Ulcer recurrence prevention during low- dose aspirin therapy

Low dose aspirin is used to prevent thrombi formation in at-risk patients. Using this treatment, however, exposes the patient to possible recurrent ulcers. Thus, it is prescribed alongside PPIs to combat this side effect. One study on 574 patients compared lansoprazole 15 mg and two Vonoprazan groups of 10 mg and 20 mg respectively.

The proportion of patients with endoscopically confirmed recurrent peptic ulcer during the 24-week treatment period (primary endpoint) was higher in the lansoprazole 15 mg group (2.8%; 6 of 213 patients) than in the vonoprazan 10 mg (0.5%; 1 of 197 patients) and vonoprazan 20 mg groups (1.5%; 3 of 196 patients). The differences in recurrence rate between the lansoprazole 15 mg group and the vonoprazan 10 mg and 20 mg groups were −2.3% and −1.3%, respectively. The non-inferiority of Vonoprazan to Lansoprazole 15 mg was verified (p < 0.001).

The differences in recurrence rates between vonoprazan 10 mg and lansoprazole 15 mg (−2.3%) and between vonoprazan 20 mg and lansoprazole 15 mg (−1.3%) were not statistically significant [23]. In conclusion, PPI or Vonoprazan are recommended for the prevention of low- dose aspirin therapy, including those with a history of ulcers or bleeding ulcers according to the Japanese guideline [3, 23].

8. Vonoprazan and gastroesophageal reflux disease (GERD)

As some patients with GERD are not controlled with their disease control under PPI, the vonoprazan therapy seems to be reasonable. In a retrospective study, GERD symptoms in the non-erosive group improved compared to baseline and remained better after 1 year of vonoprazan therapy, similar to the erosive group. Also, vonoprazan improved epigastric pain and postprandial distress symptoms in the non-erosive group and 1 year of vonoprazan therapy did not aggravate constipation or diarrhea [24]. A randomized controlled study on 73 patients with erosive esophagitis compared vonoprazan 20 mg (n = 37) or 10 mg (n = 36) for 4 weeks as the initial treatment followed by maintenance treatment with 10 mg for 8 weeks. The vonoprazan 10 mg group showed a similar therapeutic effect to the 20 mg group in mucosal healing at 4 weeks and in symptom relief throughout the study period [25]. A metaanalysis comprising six studies on this subject showed that vonoprazan is more effective than PPIs for patients with severe erosive esophagitis [26]. In the case of refractory patients, the behavioral disorders seem to be responsible for it in 20% of cases, so the high-resolution manometry, and 24-h multiluminal impedance pH-metry should be realized in such patients [27]. The level of pH should be higher than 5 for obtaining the clinical alleviation [28].

A cost-utility analysis proved that the Vonoprazan-first strategy increased quality-adjusted life years and appeared to be cost-effective for GERD patients compared with the esomeprazole- or rabeprazole-first strategies [29]. Intermittent use of Vonoprazan seems to be the most cost-efficient therapy in controlling GERD symptoms [30].

9. Conclusion

Vonoprazan has proven to be a viable and sometimes desired alternative to normal PPI treatment in case of ulcers or other circumstances that cause gastric acid imbalance. Its role in cost-efficiency analysis should be established in further studies.

Conflict of interest

The author declares no conflict of interest.

Author details

Radu Seicean[1,2]

1 "Iuliu Hațieganu" University of Medicine and Pharmacy, Cluj-Napoca, Romania

2 "Gastro Med" Medical Center, Cluj-Napoca, Romania

*Address all correspondence to: rseicean@yahoo.com

IntechOpen

References

[1] Yang X, Li Y, Sun Y, et al. Vonoprazan: A novel and potent alternative in the treatment of acid-related diseases. Digestive Diseases and Sciences. 2018;**63**:302-311. DOI: 10.1007/s10620-017-4866-6

[2] Echizen H. The first-in-class potassium-competitive acid blocker, vonoprazan fumarate: Pharmacokinetic and pharmacodynamic considerations. Clinical Pharmacokinetics. 2016;**55**(4): 409-418. DOI: 10.1007/s40262-015-0326-7

[3] Liu C, Wang Y, Shi J, Zhang C, Nie J, Li S, et al. The status and progress of first-line treatment against *Helicobacter pylori* infection: A review. Therapeutic Advances in Gastroenterology. 2021 Jun;**28**(14):1756284821989177. DOI: 10.1177/1756284821989177

[4] Ichida T, Ueyama S, Eto T, Kusano F, Sakai Y. Randomized controlled trial comparing the effects of vonoprazan plus rebamipide and esomeprazole plus rebamipide on gastric ulcer healing induced by endoscopic submucosal dissection. Internal Medicine. 2019;**58**(2):159-166. DOI: 10.2169/internalmedicine.1146-18

[5] Irai A, Takeuchi T, Takahashi Y, et al. Comparison of the effects of vonoprazan and lansoprazole for treating endoscopic submucosal dissection-induced artificial ulcers. Digestive Diseases and Sciences. 2018;**63**:974-981. DOI: 10.1007/s10620-018-4948-0

[6] Ban H, Inatomi O, Murata M, Otsuka T, Oi M, Matsumoto H, et al. Vonoprazan vs lansoprazole for the treatment of artificial gastric ulcer after endoscopic submucosal dissection: a prospective randomized comparative study. Journal of Clinical Biochemistry and Nutrition. 2021;**68**(3):259-263. DOI: 10.3164/jcbn.20-143

[7] Yamasaki A, Yoshio T, Muramatsu Y, Horiuchi Y, Ishiyama A, Hirasawa T, et al. Vonoprazan is superior to rabeprazole for healing endoscopic submucosal dissection: Induced ulcers. Digestion. 2018;**97**:170-176. DOI: 10.1159/000485028

[8] Liu C, Feng BC, Zhang Y, Li LX, Zuo XL, Li YQ. The efficacy of vonoprazan for management of post-endoscopic submucosal dissection ulcers compared with proton pump inhibitors: A meta-analysis. Journal of Digestive Diseases. 2019;**20**(10): 503-511. DOI: 10.1111/1751-2980.12813

[9] Jaruvongvanich V, Poonsombudlert K, Ungprasert P. Vonoprazan versus proton-pump inhibitors for gastric endoscopic submucosal dissection-induced ulcers: a systematic review and meta-analysis. European Journal of Gastroenterology & Hepatology. 2018;**30**(12):1416-1421. DOI: 10.1097/MEG.0000000000001204

[10] Liu C, Feng BC, Zhang Y, Li LX, Zuo XL, Li YQ. The efficacy of vonoprazan for management of post-endoscopic submucosal dissection ulcers compared with proton pump inhibitors: A meta-analysis. Journal of Digestive Diseases. 2019;**20**(10): 503-511. DOI: 10.1111/1751-2980.12813

[11] Martin ZY, Meng CX, Takagi T, Tian YS. Vonoprazan vs proton pump inhibitors in treating post-endoscopic submucosal dissection ulcers and preventing bleeding: A meta-analysis of randomized controlled trials and observational studies. Medicine (Baltimore). 2020 Feb;**99**(9):e19357. DOI: 10.1097/MD.0000000000019357

[12] He HS, Li BY, Chen QT, Song CY, Shi J, Shi B. Comparison of the use of vonoprazan and proton pump inhibitors for the treatment of peptic ulcers resulting from endoscopic submucosal

dissection: A systematic review and meta-analysis. Medical Science Monitor. 2019 Feb;**13**(25):1169-1176. DOI: 10.12659/MSM.911886

[13] Shiratori Y, Niikura R, Ishii N, Ikeya T, Honda T, Hasatani K, et al. Vonoprazan versus proton pump inhibitors for postendoscopic submucosal dissection bleeding in the stomach: A multicenter population-based comparative study. Gastrointestinal Endoscopy. 2021; **S0016-5107**(21):01479-01476. DOI: 10.1016/j.gie.2021.06.032

[14] Ishida T, Dohi O, Yamada S, Yasuda T, Yamada N, Tomie A, et al. Clinical outcomes of vonoprazan-treated patients after endoscopic submucosal dissection for gastric neoplasms: A prospective multicenter observation study. Digestion. 2021; **102**(3):386-396. DOI: 10.1159/000507807

[15] Gunaratne AW, Hamblin H, Clancy A, Magat AJMC, Dawson MVM, Tu J, et al. Combinations of antibiotics and vonoprazan for the treatment of Helicobacter pylori infections-Exploratory study. Helicobacter. 2021 Oct;**26**(5):e12830. DOI: 10.1111/hel.12830

[16] Suzuki S, Gotoda T, Kusano C, Ikehara H, Ichijima R, Ohyauchi M, et al. Seven-day vonoprazan and low-dose amoxicillin dual therapy as first-line *Helicobacter pylori* treatment: a multicentrerandomised trial in Japan. Gut. Jun 2020;**69**(6):1019-1026. DOI: 10.1136/gutjnl-2019-319954

[17] Rokkas T, Gisbert JP, Malfertheiner P, Niv Y, Gasbarrini A, Leja M, et al. Comparative effectiveness of multiple different first-line treatment regimens for helicobacter pylori infection: A network meta-analysis. Gastroenterology. 2021;**161**(2): 495-507.e4. DOI: 10.1053/j.gastro.2021.04.012

[18] Kamada T, Satoh K, Itoh T, Ito M, Iwamoto J, Okimoto T, et al. Evidence-based clinical practice guidelines for peptic ulcer disease 2020. Journal of Gastroenterology. 2021;**56**(4):303-322. DOI: 10.1007/s00535-021-01769-0

[19] Lyu QJ, Pu QH, Zhong XF, Zhang J. Efficacy and safety of vonoprazan-based versus proton pump inhibitor-based triple therapy for *Helicobacter pylori* eradication: A meta-analysis of randomized clinical trials. BioMed Research International. 2019;**2019**: 9781212. DOI: 10.1155/2019/9781212

[20] Eto H, Suzuki S, Kusano C, Ikehara H, Ichijima R, Ito H, et al. Impact of body size on first-line Helicobacter pylori eradication success using vonoprazan and amoxicillin dual therapy. Helicobacter. 2021;**26**(2): e12788. DOI: 10.1111/hel.12788

[21] Suzuki S, Gotoda T, Takano C, Horii T, Sugita T, Ogura K, et al. Long term impact of vonoprazan-based Helicobacter pylori treatment on gut microbiota and its relation to post-treatment body weight changes. Helicobacter. Dec 2021;**26**(6):e12851. DOI: 10.1111/hel.12851. Epub 2021 Sep 6. PMID: 34486195

[22] Mizokami Y, Oda K, Funao N, Nishimura A, Soen S, Kawai T, et al. Vonoprazan prevents ulcer recurrence during long-term NSAID therapy: Randomised, lansoprazole-controlled non-inferiority and single-blind extension study. Gut. 2018;**67**(6):1042-1051. DOI: 10.1136/gutjnl-2017-314010. Epub 2017 Oct 7

[23] Kawai T, Oda K, Funao N, Nishimura A, Matsumoto Y, Mizokami Y, et al. Vonoprazan prevents low-dose aspirin-associated ulcer recurrence: Randomised phase 3 study. Gut. 2018;**67**(6):1033-1041. DOI: 10.1136/gutjnl-2017-314852. Epub 2017 Dec 1

[24] Shinozaki S, Osawa H, Hayashi Y, Miura Y, Lefor AK, Yamamoto H.

Long-term vonoprazan therapy is effective for controlling symptomatic proton pump inhibitor-resistant gastroesophageal reflux disease. Biomed Rep. 2021;**14**(3):32. DOI: 10.3892/br.2021

[25] Okanobu H, Kohno T, Mouri R, Hatsushika Y, Yamashita Y, Miyaki E, et al. Efficacy of vonoprazan 10 mg compared with 20 mg for the initial treatment in patients with erosive esophagitis: A randomized pilot study. Esophagus. 2021;**18**(3):669-675. DOI: 10.1007/s10388-020-00798-7

[26] Cheng Y, Liu J, Tan X, Dai Y, Xie C, Li X, et al. Direct comparison of the efficacy and safety of vonoprazan versus proton-pump inhibitors for gastroesophageal reflux disease: A systematic review and meta-analysis. Digestive Diseases and Sciences. 2021;**66**(1):19-28. DOI: 10.1007/s10620-020-06141-5

[27] Hoshikawa Y, Hoshino S, Kawami N, Iwakiri K. Prevalence of behavioral disorders in patients with vonoprazan-refractory reflux symptoms. Journal of Gastroenterology. 2021 Feb;**56**(2):117-124. DOI: 10.1007/s00535-020-01751-2

[28] Abe Y, Koike T, Saito M, Okata T, Nakagawa K, Hatta W, et al. The ameliorating effect of switching to vonoprazan: A novel potassium-competitive acid blocker in patients with proton pump inhibitor refractory non-erosive reflux disease. Digestion. 2021;**102**(3):480-488. DOI: 10.1159/000506152

[29] Yokoya Y, Igarashi A, Uda A, Deguchi H, Takeuchi T, Higuchi K. Cost-utility analysis of a 'vonoprazan-first' strategy versus 'esomeprazole- or rabeprazole-first' strategy in GERD. Journal of Gastroenterology. 2019; **54**(12):1083-1095. DOI: 10.1007/s00535-019-01609-2

[30] Habu Y, Hamasaki R, Maruo M, Nakagawa T, Aono Y, Hachimine D. Treatment strategies for reflux esophagitis including a potassium-competitive acid blocker: A cost-effectiveness analysis in Japan. J Gen Fam Med. 2021;**22**(5):237-245. DOI: 10.1002/jgf2.429